About the Editors

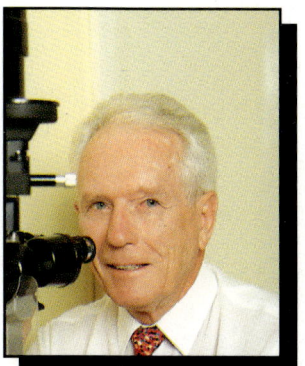

Dr Paul Moffitt

❏ Dr Paul Moffitt conceived and instituted the first Diabetes Education and Stabilisation Centre in Australia. He was Director until he commenced private consulting practice in Newcastle during 1989 and is Clinical Associate Professor of Medicine at the University of Newcastle.

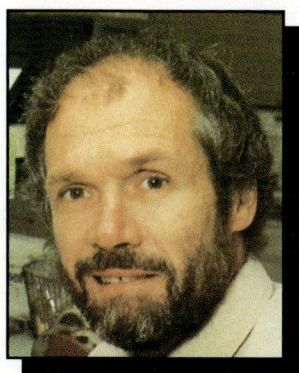

Dr Pat Phillips

❏ Dr Pat Phillips is Director of the Endocrine and Diabetes Service, The Queen Elizabeth Hospital, Adelaide. He is chair of the Health Care and Education Committee of Diabetes Australia, Secretary of the Australian Diabetes Society and a member of the NH & MRC Expert Panel on Diabetes.

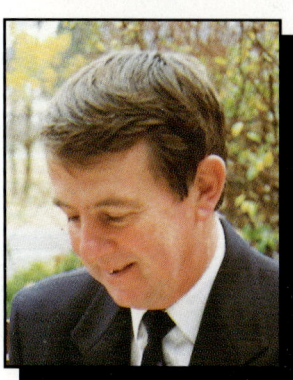

Bernie Ayers

❏ Bernie Ayers joined the National Office of Diabetes Australia in 1989 as Director, Health Promotion & Research. He was previously National Director, Health Promotion for the Department of Health, Housing and Community Services in Canberra. Bernie also spent a year in Denmark as a consultant to the World Health Organisation on health promotion. He is also Secretary to the NH & MRC Expert Panel on Diabetes.

DIABETES & YOU –
AN OWNER'S MANUAL

Foreword

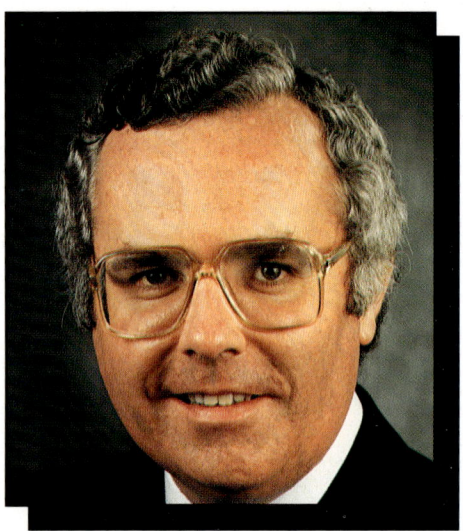

*E*very so often a book comes along and instantly assumes a "state of the art" mantle in its field. **Diabetes and You – An Owner's Manual** is such a book. I use it regularly as a reference. The first edition sold over 10,000 copies. This second edition will no doubt be just as popular.

It is a very special book because it brings together the most knowledgeable experts on diabetes in Australia. These 30 authors are well known in this country and most have made their mark on the international diabetes scene.

The book would not have happened without the generous contributions of these dedicated authors and on behalf of Diabetes Australia, I would like to thank them.

A special note of thanks needs to go to the editors as well. They have done a marvellous job in bringing all the contributions together into a very readable book.

This is the first in the series of four Diabetes and You publications. The others in the series — Living with Insulin, All About Type 2 Diabetes and an eight module card series — are available from Diabetes Australia.

Special mention must also be made of the generosity of Lilly Diabetes Care in sponsoring the Diabetes & You series.

The book is full of important information. Once read, this book will also become an invaluable reference and a vital partner to all those Australians who have diabetes, their families and their friends, as well as the health professionals who care for them.

Terry Sheahan
National President
Diabetes Australia

Contents

INTRODUCTION

1. Diabetes – What goes wrong 1
2. Types of Diabetes 5
3. Living with Diabetes 8

MANAGEMENT AND LIFESTYLE

4. Diabetes and Lifestyle 11
5. Diet and Diabetes 15
6. The Use of Tablets 21

INSULIN AND MONITORING

7. Insulin and Its Role 25
8. Injections and Injectors 32
9. Self Monitoring of Blood Glucose 39
10. Testing Urine 46
11. Hypoglycaemia and Hyperglycaemia 51
12. Diabetes and Exercise 56
13. Sick Days 62
14. Diabetes and Other Medications 68

COMPLICATIONS

15. Chronic Complications of Diabetes 75
16. Diabetes and Eyes 81
17. Caring for Feet 86
18. Diabetes and Pregnancy 89
19. Diabetes and Female Sexuality 95
20. Sexual Problems in Men 96
21. You and Your Health care Team 99

SPECIAL GROUPS

22. The Schoolchild with Diabetes 105
23. Diabetes – A Problem in any Language ... 110
24. Diabetes in Aborigines 112

SOCIAL ISSUES

25. Rights and Responsibilities 117
26. Insurance and Diabetes 120
27. Travel 123
28. Further Resources 132

SPECIAL ISSUES

29. The Genetics of Diabetes 135
30. Progress in Diabetes Research 139

Glossary 143

Index 148

Abbreviations and measures 151

DIABETES & YOU
An owner's manual

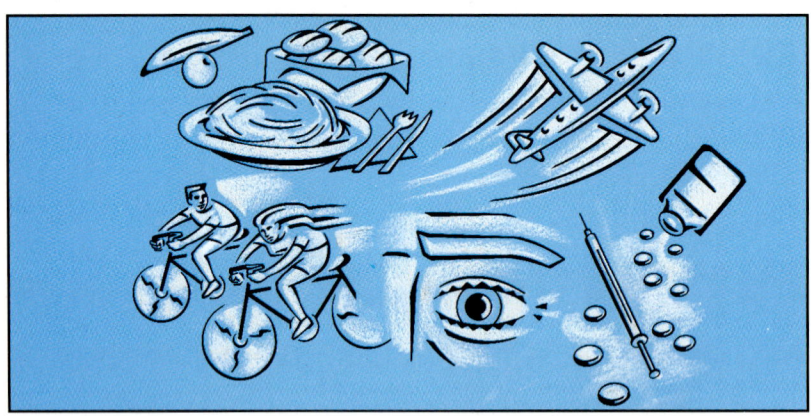

INTRODUCTION

❏ Diabetes – What Goes Wrong?

What's in a name
A question of balance
Where does glucose come from?
Insulin enters the story
Maintaining the balance
What are you aiming for?
Controlling diabetes

❏ Types of Diabetes

Who gets diabetes, and how?
How is it diagnosed?
How is it treated?
Can diabetes be cured?
Where to get help and information
Knowledge is power

❏ Living With Diabetes

Team Effort
Understand your diabetes
We have come a long way

CHAPTER 1

Diabetes – What goes wrong?

By Dr Pat Phillips,
Director, Endocrine and Diabetes Service
The Queen Elizabeth Hospital
Adelaide, SA

Diabetes was known in ancient times. In fact, the name 'Diabetes' comes from the Greek::
Dia = through
betes = a passing
This refers to the "passing through" the body of large volumes of fluid. The full name "Diabetes Mellitus" refers to sweetness (mellitus = honey). The sweetness of the urine and body fluids is because of too much sugar. This is the basic problem in diabetes.

Your body needs a special sugar, glucose. Your body makes glucose from starchy foods (carbohydrates like bread, potatoes) and other sugars (like sucrose – table sugar, fructose – fruit sugar). The glucose is carried around the body in the blood and the level is called "glycaemia" (glyc = glucose; aemia = in the blood).

A Question of Balance

Your glucose level must be "not too high .... not too low .... but just right".

A high level (*hyperglycaemia*) affects the body's machinery.
– Things don't work as well. You feel tired and sleepy.
– The body fluids are concentrated and the lens in your eye changes shape. You get blurry vision.
– The kidneys filtering the blood collect more glucose than usual. This glucose must be carried out of the body. You pass a lot of urine (polyuria; poly = lots and uria = urine). You need more water, get thirsty and drink a lot (polydipsia; dipsia = drink).
– Your body is losing glucose from food products. You lose weight, feel hungry and eat more (polyphagia; phagia = to eat).

A low level (*hypoglycaemia*) also affects the body. Especially the brain which relies on glucose.
– Your brain doesn't like being starved of glucose. It sends urgent signals to the body. You feel hungry.
– Your brain doesn't work properly. You don't think straight. You get trembly.

HYPER'S AND HYPO'S

Hyperglycaemia = high blood glucose levels
Hypoglycaemia = low blood glucose levels

THE POLY'S

Polyuria = passing lots of urine
Polydipsia = drinking lots of fluid
Polyphagia = eating lots of food

Controlling diabetes is keeping the balance "just right".

Where does glucose come from?

The meals you eat have:
- Protein – for body growth and repair
- Fat – lots of concentrated calories
- Carbohydrate – starchy foods and sugars. Each is made up of *simple* units. Starch has hundreds of smaller units joined together. It's a *complex* carbohydrate.

The smaller units in starch are sugars (like glucose, fructose). They are *simple* carbohydrates.

Diabetes – What Goes Wrong

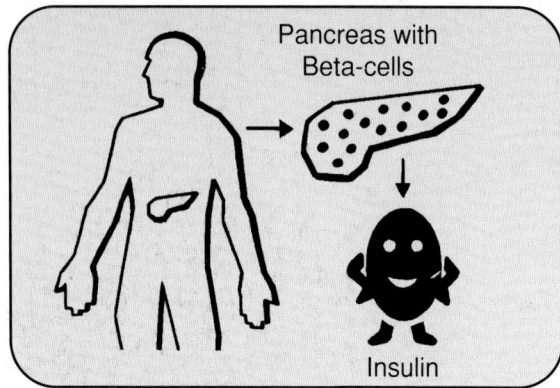

Diagram 1

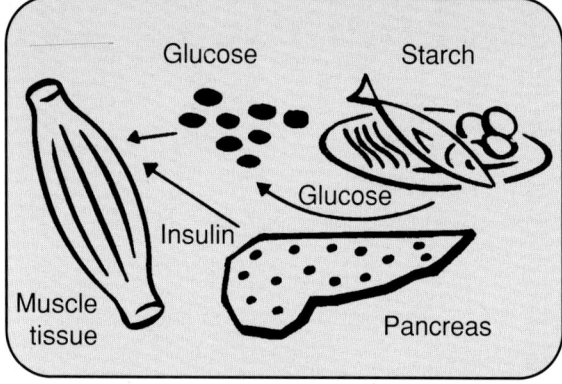

Diagram 2

Your food is broken down by digestive juices. Starch is digested into sugars which the liver makes into glucose.

Your body can't change straw into gold (remember the fairy-tale of Rumplestiltskin), but it can change bread into glucose!

Insulin enters the story

Now you have changed starch into glucose racing around in the blood stream. But the glucose has to get out of the blood and into the body tissues. It's the cells in the body tissues that actually do the work. Brain cells so you can think, heart cells so you can pump blood, muscle cells so you can walk.

Insulin opens the doors (the glucose channels) that let glucose go from the blood to the body cells.

Insulin comes from the pancreas, which is a gland sitting just below the stomach – half way between your tummy button and the line joining your nipples. Most of the cells of the pancreas make digestive juices, but some cells (the beta cells) make insulin which travels in the blood and tells the food products where to go (Diagram 1 & 2).

Maintaining the balance

Your body is very clever. A high blood glucose level makes the pancreas put out more insulin. Insulin opens the glucose channels and glucose goes from the blood into the cells. The glucose level falls. The body gets back into balance.

At rest, the cells don't need much glucose. The glucose channels are difficult to open and there is not much insulin (Diagram 3).

After a meal containing starch, blood glucose increases. The pancreas releases insulin. Insulin opens glucose channels and the cells use the glucose (Diagram 4).

With exercise, muscle cells need glucose. There is not much insulin, but glucose channels become easy to open and allow enough glucose through (Diagram 5).

In diabetes, the insulin levels are decreased or insulin does not work properly. Glucose channels are shut. Glucose builds up in the blood and causes problems (Diagram 6).

The balancing act

The aim of diabetes treatment, is to keep the blood glucose balanced in the normal range. In diabetes, this is no longer done automatically by the body. People with diabetes must organise and juggle food and stress, insulin/tablets and exercise. They balance:
- The things that raise blood glucose – food and stress
- The things that lower blood glucose – exercise and insulin/tablets.

If this balancing act is successful, blood glucose doesn't go too high (hyper), or too low (hypo), but stays in the healthy range (Diagram 7).

Highs and lows

Glucose levels go up and down through the day.

"LOWS" (low blood glucose) occur before

Living with Diabetes

meals, after exercise and sometimes in the middle of the night when there is a long gap between meals.

"HIGHS" (high blood glucose) occur about two hours after meals and when you are under stress.

Blood glucose is measured in millimoles of glucose per litre of blood (mmol/L).

A normal blood glucose level is 5mmol/L and is equivalent to about one sixth of a teaspoon of glucose per litre of blood.

What are you aiming for?

The basic problem with diabetes is that the blood glucose level rises. This abnormal chemistry can damage the body. It is important to control blood glucose to avoid problems.

Everyone is different. You and your health care team will work out your own personal goals. In a perfect world, we would aim at the levels which occur in people without diabetes because we believe that this minimises long-term problems. Often though, it is impossible to get this ideal control and trying too hard, causes blood glucose swings from HI to LO!

It is a question of finding the balance which suits you best.

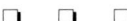

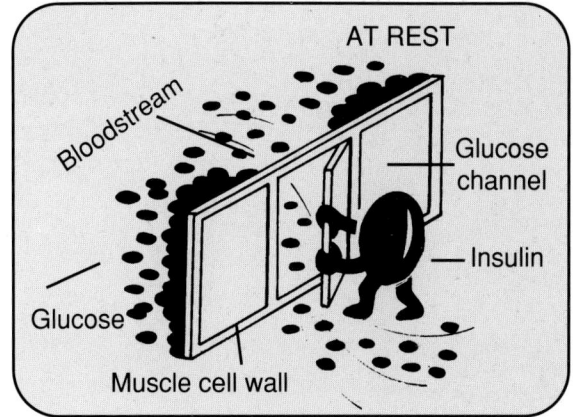

Diagram 3

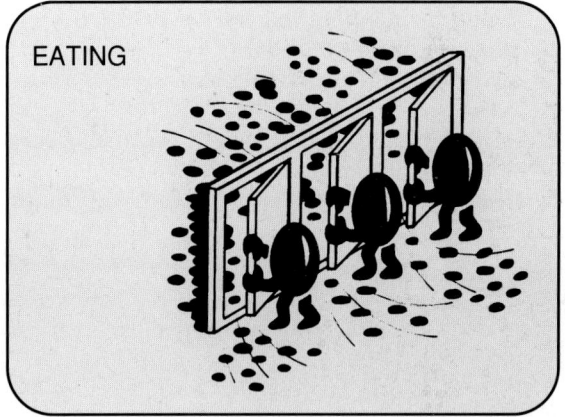

Diagram 4

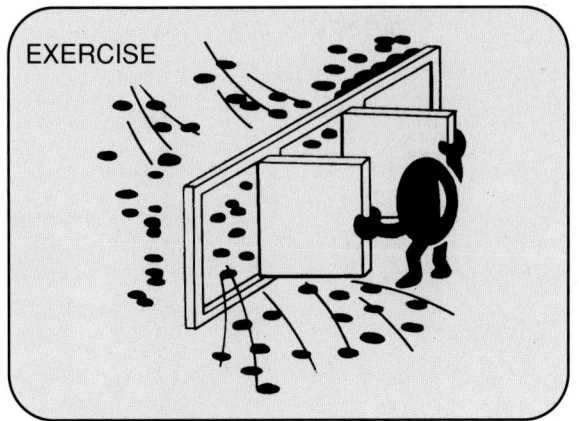

Diagram 5

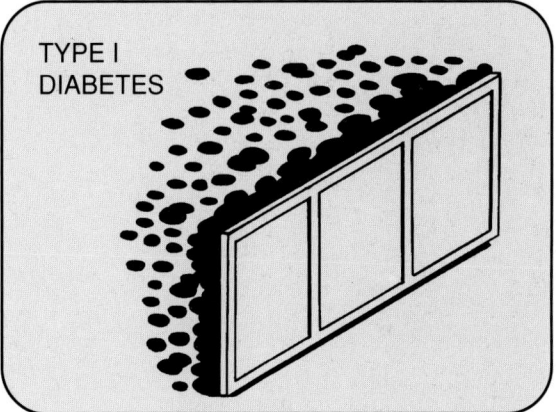

Diagram 6

Diabetes – What Goes Wrong

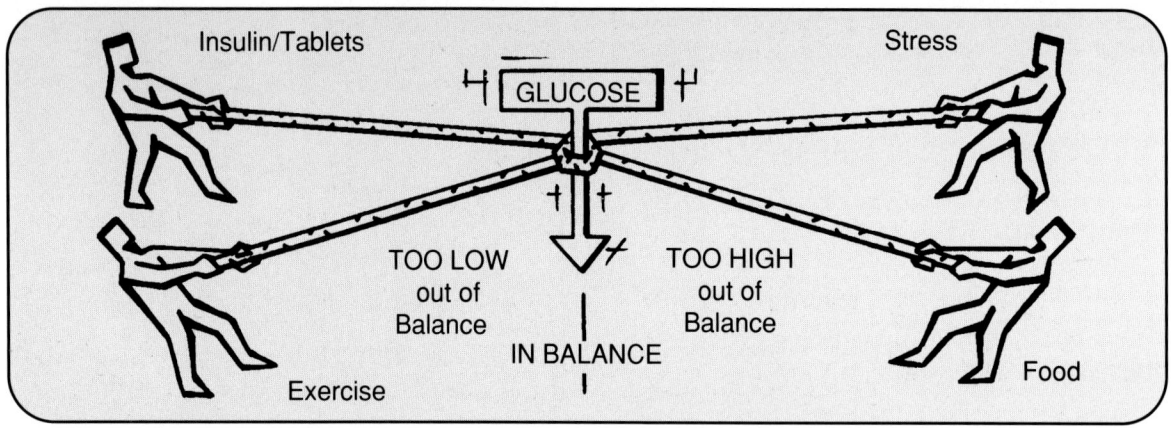

Diagram 7

Controlling diabetes

In future chapters you will see the three steps to balancing glucose levels:
1. **A healthy diet providing glucose at the right rate.**
2. **Regular exercise and weight control to keep glucose channels in good shape.**
3. **Tablets or insulin if needed, to boost insulin supply or activity.**

To take these three steps you need:

- **A healthy life-style** – diabetes control is based on the "golden guides" for a healthy life-style.
- **A team approach** – you, your family and your health professionals, are a team working together to find the best way for you to live with your diabetes.

CHAPTER 2

Types of Diabetes

By Dr Tony V. Stepanas
Senior Specialist Endocrinologist
Royal Canberra Hospital
Canberra

Diabetes is a disease in which the body is unable to properly use its main fuel, glucose – a form of sugar.

This happens if the pancreas, a gland which lies behind the stomach, is unable to make enough insulin, or the insulin it makes is unable to work effectively. Insulin is a hormone which normally circulates in the blood. It helps glucose to get inside the body's cells. The glucose is then used as a fuel to allow the cells to do whatever job they do, such as a heart muscle cell to beat, a nerve cell to feel pain.

Without insulin, glucose cannot enter the body's cells, it builds up in the blood, spills out into the urine, and, if not treated, can seriously damage the body.

There are two main types of diabetes:
- Type 1 or Insulin Dependent Diabetes, which usually develops in young people but is fairly uncommon, accounting for about one in every five cases of diabetes.
- Type 2 or Non Insulin Dependent Diabetes, which usually develops in overweight people over 40 years of age. It is more common, accounting for about four out of every five cases of diabetes.

Who gets diabetes and how?

About half a million – or three out of every one hundred Australians have diabetes. Anyone can develop it at any age although the majority of people with diabetes are born with a susceptibility to develop it.

Type 1 (insulin dependent) diabetes can be brought on by a viral infection which damages the pancreas beyond repair, resulting in complete insulin deficiency.

In the case of Type 2 (non insulin dependent) diabetes, being overweight, unfit, stressed or simply getting older, may lead to insulin not working properly and the eventual "exhaustion" of the pancreas.

There are three common misconceptions about diabetes:
- Diabetes is not a contagious disease: you cannot "catch it".
- Diabetes is not caused by eating too much sugar.
- Although easy to treat, Type 2 diabetes is not a "mild" form of diabetes. If not properly treated, it can have serious consequences.

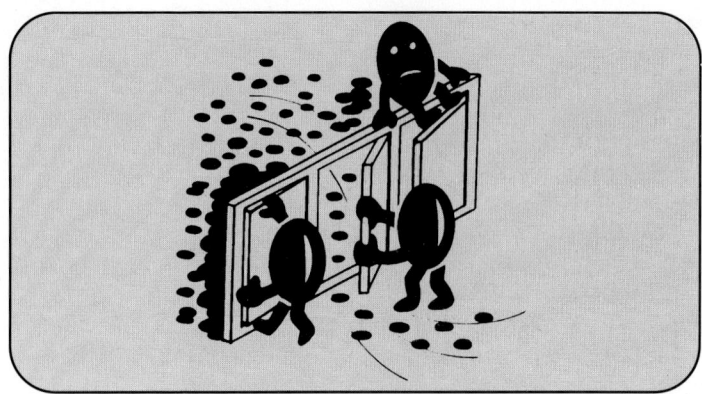

In Type 2 diabetes insulin does not work properly and the insulin channels are difficult to open.

How is diabetes diagnosed?

The typical symptoms of diabetes are as follows but they need not all be present in the one person:
- Increased urination
- Increased thirst

Types of Diabetes

- Tiredness and a lack of energy
- Weight loss or, in some cases, weight gain
- Skin infections and itching, especially genital
- Blurred vision

Symptoms may develop quickly (in days or weeks) in someone with Type 1 diabetes, or slowly (in months or years) in Type 2 diabetes.

A doctor must be seen if two or more of these symptoms are present. A blood test showing a high glucose level will then confirm the diagnosis.

Up to half the patients with Type 2 diabetes may have no obvious symptoms: a high blood or urine glucose level may be found on a routine medical check. An overweight person with vague ill health should be checked for diabetes, especially if they have relatives with diabetes.

How is diabetes treated?

Proper treatment of diabetes depends on adopting a healthy lifestyle. That is, a healthy, balanced diet high in fibre (roughage) and low in fat and sweet foods, and regular exercise.

In those who are at risk of developing Type 2 diabetes, this is also the way to delay or prevent its development.

The diagnosis of diabetes will mean changes to lifestyle, there is no way around that but there is no reason why the person with diabetes cannot continue to lead a normal, active life. A new routine will have to be established but through a working understanding of the disease, this routine can be tailored to fit in with normal everyday life.

Basically, people with Type 1 diabetes will need to take regular insulin injections while those with Type 2 diabetes might need tablets. After many years, some might even need insulin injections.

All must check control of their diabetes by regularly self-testing glucose levels in the blood or urine.

Diabetes is not a barrier to a happy, fulfilling life. Many people learn to live successfully with diabetes in all walks of life, including sporting heroes, politicians, manual workers, business people, media and entertainment personalities.

However allowances have to be made,

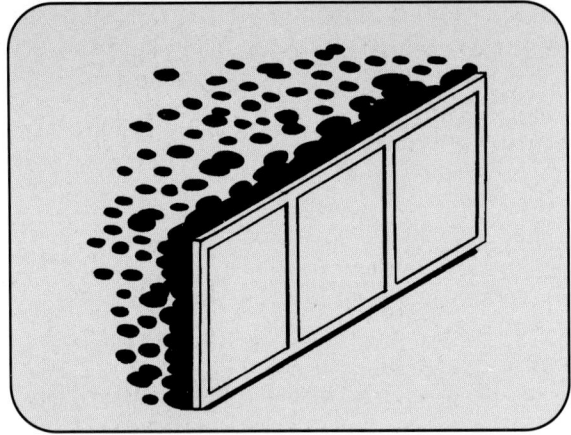

In Type 1 diabetes there is no insulin and the glucose channels are shut

especially with Type 1 diabetes, for certain type of jobs, vigorous sports and long distance travel. Authorities such as drivers' licence departments and insurance companies will have to be notified. It is essential to stop smoking and wise to limit alcohol. Some medicines have to be selected more carefully by the doctor of pharmacist.

Poorly controlled diabetes can cause complications. Very low or very high blood glucose levels cause unpleasant symptoms. After many years, poorly controlled diabetes might damage the eyes, nerves, kidneys and arteries.

The key is knowledge. All people with diabetes must learn as much as they can about the disease and its treatment and ensure regular follow-up with their doctor, diabetes educator, dietitian and other members of the health care team.

Can diabetes be cured?

No. There is no cure for diabetes yet, but it can be controlled by peoples' own efforts at following their treatment routine.

Where to get help and information about diabetes

Most big city hospitals have diabetes clinics run by diabetes specialists and many country hospitals and community nursing centres also have clinics run by diabetes educators in conjunction with local doctors.

Types of Diabetes

DIABETES AUSTRALIA is a registered, charitable organisation looking after the needs of all those with diabetes and all those dealing with diabetes. It has a wide network of branches in each state and territory, with headquarters in each capital city.

❏ ❏ ❏

Knowledge is power

As we have said, the key to managing your diabetes and living a full and happy life is knowledge. People with diabetes must always be seeking information about their diabetes. The more they know, the more easily they will handle any situation.

This book is aimed at providing information, but by no means should it be the end of the quest for knowledge. Always be prepared to discuss your situation with the professional people who make up the diabetes health care team.

Above all, do not feel guilty if you do not understand any particular aspect of diabetes or its treatment. Remember: always ask as many questions as you need until you are perfectly satisfied with the answers – this is the only way you will gain the confidence needed to control your diabetes.

Never has the saying "knowledge is power" been more true than in the personal control of diabetes. With knowledge comes confidence, with confidence comes the ability to control your diabetes – and not have it control you..

CHAPTER 3

Living with Diabetes

By Ian McEwen
Past National President, Diabetes Australia

Succeeding in life with diabetes is like winning the Cox Plate – Australia's championship in the thoroughbred world. To win the Cox Plate you need the absolute in team effort on the part of trainer, jockey and horse. To make a success of your life with diabetes you need that same team effort from you the patient, the doctor, the allied health professionals and a fourth element, your family.

My 40 years with diabetes has been that team effort.

I go back to 1951 when the diabetes specialist of the day at Wellington Hospital in New Zealand told me on discharge from two week's stabilisation: "You're young, you appear intelligent and now that we have your diabetes under control, study this book – Dr Lawrence's The Diabetic Life – learn to treat yourself, keep in touch with your doctor and look after your body."

That advice is as good today as it was then. In fact, it is the best possible advice I can pass on to any person with diabetes, young or old.

Getting to understand your diabetes is a matter of learning, reading all the literature you can from Diabetes Australia or any other source – but remember, it must be authoritative, not listening to other people's experiences or reading of them. There is enough information about diabetes today to give you a very wide choice and this book provides an excellent starting point whether you take insulin or diet and tablets.

For example, not only must you learn about your daily food intake, you must also learn about care of your feet, your skin, your eyes. You must learn to recognise any change in your body functions or appearance. That is where the doctor and health professionals come into your life.

Care of the feet is particularly important. My podiatrist tells me my feet are better than many of his patients who do not have diabetes. I achieve this by daily washing, daily application of cream, six-weekly visits to the podiatrist and wearing comfortable shoes and socks.

Diet is often a problem. So often I hear diabetic friends say: "I can't eat this or that." Sure you can't, but a negative attitude does not help you learn to live with diabetes. If you want a piece of cake, one small piece really won't hurt as long as you remember at your next meal that you have had it. One small piece is not plural. After a hard day's work in the garden, a refreshing glass of beer is not going to ruin a diet, but it must be just one.

This all leads to a complete understanding of your daily intake of food, understanding what your diet is, what it contains and what effect it has on you. In the old days, "substitutes" were common, today the technology is the same but you should be able to understand what you are substituting for what.

In my busy life at Moonee Valley, which means extended working hours, extensive social activities and an expanded lifestyle, I have always coped with blending the requirements of diabetes with my job. I do not see myself as an exception – just a practical application of one problem to another – and I have no hesitation in telling anyone I have diabetes. In my four daily injections schedule, my NovoPen is as common at every dining room table as the knife and fork.

Development of a four times a day injection schedule was accomplished with my specialist, with whom I have been consulting for my 20 years in Australia, every six months without fail or more often when the need has arisen.

I have found injections with every meal gives me comfortable control. It was not always like that but the refinements in the manufacture of insulin and the production of human insulin have certainly been very beneficial. This is not to say that it is the ideal schedule for everyone but it highlights the fact that taking insulin can be varied to suit your needs – it should not be your master.

I have seen many changes in treating diabetes over the past 40 years. In the early 1950s almost every ounce of food was weighed before consumption. Insulin was taken once a day by glass syringe with needles that were seldom sharp. Urine testing was by boiling up Benedict's solution which often exploded from a test tube. The alternative to the rigid diet was carbohydrate-free food like rhubarb or gluten rolls. There was not even sugar-free chewing gum.

❏ ❏ ❏

The comparison today says we have come a long way in making the life of the person with diabetes more comfortable. Blood glucose meters, human insulin, single use syringes, a more lenient approach to a huge variety of food and sugar free foods.

But all this does not replace the prime fundamental: the theme for the first National Diabetes Week of the decade – Eat Well, Play Well, Stay Well. Sensible eating is a good diet, sensible exercise is essential and having done these two things, you are bound to stay well.

DIABETES & YOU
An owner's manual

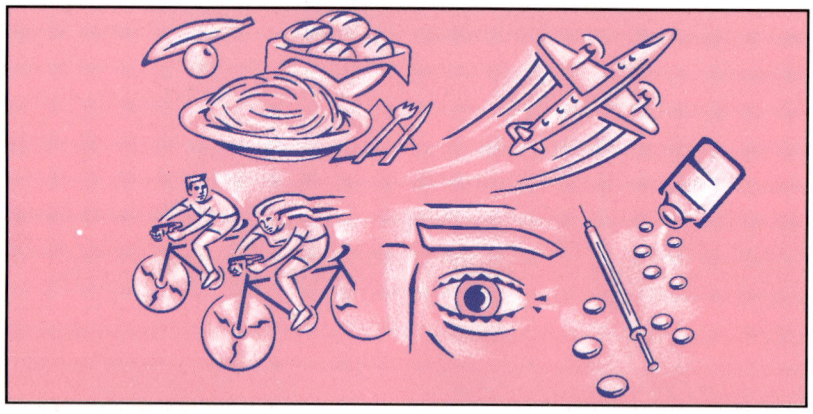

MANAGEMENT AND LIFESTYLE

❏ Diabetes and Lifestyle

Eight Golden Guidelines:
– Don't get fat
– Don't eat fat
– Eat complex carbohydrate
– Spread complex carbohydrate
– Take 30
– Take time out
– Quit for life
– Four men and women two

❏ Diet and Diabetes

Which foods are the right goods
Carbohydrates in your diet
Fibre
Blood glucose response
Proteins
Hints for reducing fat

Alcohol and diabetes
Surviving in the supermarket
Dining out
Menu suggestions
Food choice list

❏ The Use of Tablets

Tablets no substitute to diet
Effectiveness
Side Effects
Tablets when ill

CHAPTER 4

Diabetes and Lifestyle

By Pat Phillips, Director, Endocrine & Diabetes Service
The Queen Elizabeth Hospital, Adelaide, SA
and
Lynette Brown, Clinical Dietitian
Royal Canberra Hospital, Canberra, ACT

We hear a lot about diabetes and lifestyle, such adages as "Eat Well, Play Well, Stay Well" – the theme of Diabetes Week 1990, or the old saying "Type 2 diabetes is a lifestyle disease."

So why is lifestyle so important in regards to diabetes?

The short answer is that our bodies are designed as hunter-gatherers and over the centuries our lifestyle has changed. We are built to hunt wild animals and fish for their lean meat, collect fresh fruit, nuts and vegetables and gather and cook grains.

The bodies of our ancestors adapted to the high activity of hunting and gathering, and the low fat, low sugar food which were the products of that hunting and gathering.

But we have come a long way since the Stone Age. We now live in the "lucky country", an affluent society where few go hungry.

The down side of this richness is that the way we live does not suit our bodies. Our lifestyle has changed but our bodies have not. Cars, buses and bicycles mean less activity and farm bred meats and fried and sweet foods mean more fat and sugar.

Norm of the Life, Be In It television advertisement may like to sit watching TV having a beer and snacking on chips, but the effects are unhealthy.

This applies to all Australians and it applies especially if you have diabetes. Whether you have Type 1 or Type 2 diabetes, it is important to follow some rules – known as the **Eight Golden Guidelines For Lifestyle**. These are:

- **Don't get fat.** Stay trim, taut and terrific. After all, the less extra fat your body has, the better it will respond to insulin.

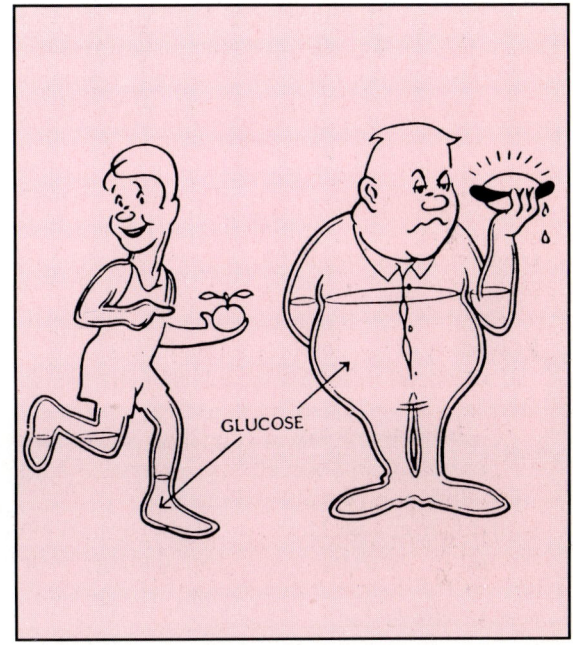

- **Don't eat fat.** Fat has lots of energy you may not need, and fat may block your blood vessels.
- **Eat complex carbohydrate.** Fruit, vegetables and cereals all have starch – complex carbohydrate, and only small amounts of the sugars which increase blood glucose levels.
- **Spread your complex carbohydrate.** Spreading food throughout the day spreads the load and gives a smooth, steady supply of glucose.
- **Take 30.** Thirty minutes of moderate activity a day has been shown to help insulin work and help your blood vessels stay healthy.
- **Take Time Out.** Stress is a real problem for everyone in today's society, but particularly for people with diabetes. Once again we can

Diabetes and Lifestyle

look back at the way our body was designed for the hunter gatherer lifestyle. Stress affects our bodies today the same way as danger affected our early forebears. When danger threatens we can either fight or take flight. Our bodies get ready – our breathing deepens, giving us more oxygen, our heart speeds up providing more blood to the muscles, our glucose stores are released to provide energy and our muscles tense, ready to fight or run. This is fine for Stone Age man, but bad news for the modern person with diabetes. The last thing you want is for your glucose stores to be released – your body has enough problems keeping glucose stored in the right place without stress pushing it out again.

Nowadays there is no way of avoiding stress, but you can help your body deal with it.

Regular activity is one way and it helps to keep your weight and blood vessels healthy as well.

Another way is to take time out for yourself. You are a pretty important person remember, and you need to look after yourself. Of course there are lots of other ways to help your body cope with stress. Look in your local newspaper for courses or in your library for books. And ask your doctor or diabetes educator.

- **Quit for life.** The labels on cigarette packets are right – smoking really does damage your health. This is true for everyone, but especially people with diabetes.

Cigarette smoke is a mixture of stimulants like nicotine which affect the brain and give a "buzz". Unfortunately these same stimulants affect blood vessels in both the short term – by closing up the walls, and the long term – by blocking off the vessels. Also cigarette smoke has carbon monoxide which stops your blood carrying oxygen.

Add this to the fact that diabetes also damages blood vessels and it is easy to see that smokers with diabetes have "double trouble" – and that's not even counting the other ill effects of cigarettes on lungs, skin, breath, eyes, kidney and last but not least, your pocket.

If you do not smoke you have lots of reasons not to smoke. If you do smoke, you have lots of reasons to give up – the best one being that you will feel so much better for it.

Drink wise – Four Men & Women Two.

This little slogan refers to standard drinks which contain 10 grams of alcohol – 300ml of beer, 100 ml of wine. In moderation, that is four drinks for men and two for women, alcohol is pleasant, sociable and safe. However it can cause three special problems for people with diabetes:

- Overweight – alcohol has lots of energy you may not need if you are trying to control your weight.
- Loss of judgement – alcohol can impair your ability to make rational decisions concerning food and medication and this can prove costly.
- Low blood glucose – just as stress releases glucose stores, alcohol can block the release and cause low blood glucose.

Generally alcohol should be taken with food. Most drinks are suitable or can be made suitable, but some have lots of sugar and are best avoided.

So there you have your **Eight Golden Guidelines**. All very well, but the real test is putting them into practice. Here's how:

Don't get fat. Measure your height in stockinged feet, in metres, such as 5ft 10in = 180 cms = 1.8 metres, and your weight in ordinary clothes in kilograms, such as 176 lbs = 13 stone 2 lbs = 81 kgs.

Diabetes and Lifestyle

To calculate your body mass index, or BMI, multiply your height by itself (1.8 x 1.8 = 3.24) and divide this into your weight (80 by 3.24 = BMI of 25)

The healthy range is 20 -25, overweight is 25 - 30 and very overweight is more than 30.

If you do need to lose weight, see your doctor, diabetes nurse or dietitian for expert advice.

Don't eat fat. Keep a food diary and write down everything you eat for one week.

Now check for fatty foods. Consider trying the alternative food choices. Make the healthy choice the easy choice, and stop buying and cooking fatty foods.

Eat complex carbohydrate and spread your complex carbohydrate. Check your food diary. Do you have a lot of sugar or sugary foods? Once more, consider alternatives.

If you don't have starchy food every time you eat, consider spreading the starch more evenly.

Take 30. Consider simple ways to increase your activity – use stairs instead of elevators, perform housework and shopping at a brisk pace, go walking during your lunch break.

Take Time Out. Put aside part of the day which you can call your own and do something you want to do. Decide on a time and stick to it.

Find out more about relaxation. Go to the council, the library, or ask your doctor or diabetes nurse.

Quit for Life. Talk to your doctor or diabetes nurse. Enquire about self help groups at your council or community health centre.

Set a date. Persuade your partner to stop too, ask friends and family to give moral support. Think about situations where you will be tempted and work out how to deal with them.

Drink Wise – Four men and Women Two. Once again make the decision. Work out times you will be tempted to take an alcoholic drink and how you will deal with the situation – or avoid it for a while.

❏ ❏ ❏

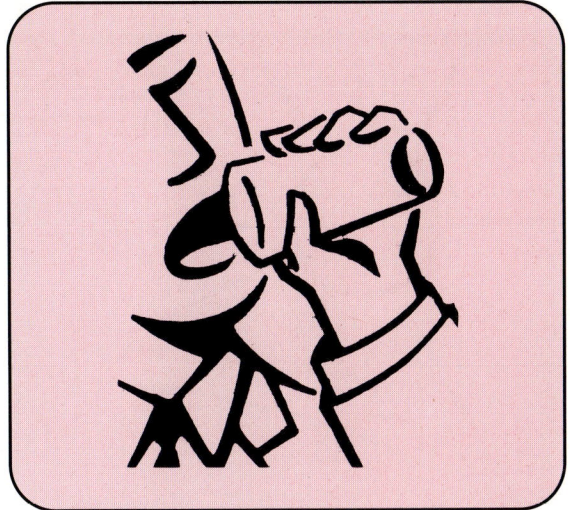

Limit alcohol – remember four drinks for men and for women two.

With all these guidelines, don't worry if you make mistakes. Keep at it and it will work out.

Remember, lifestyle is important for people with diabetes. We can't go back to the Stone Age – and we wouldn't want to, but we can keep our bodies healthy through low fat, low sugar foods, regular activity, managing everyday stress, avoiding cigarettes and moderating alcohol.

The best way of living with diabetes is to live a healthy lifestyle. This will help you and the rest of your family get the most out of life.

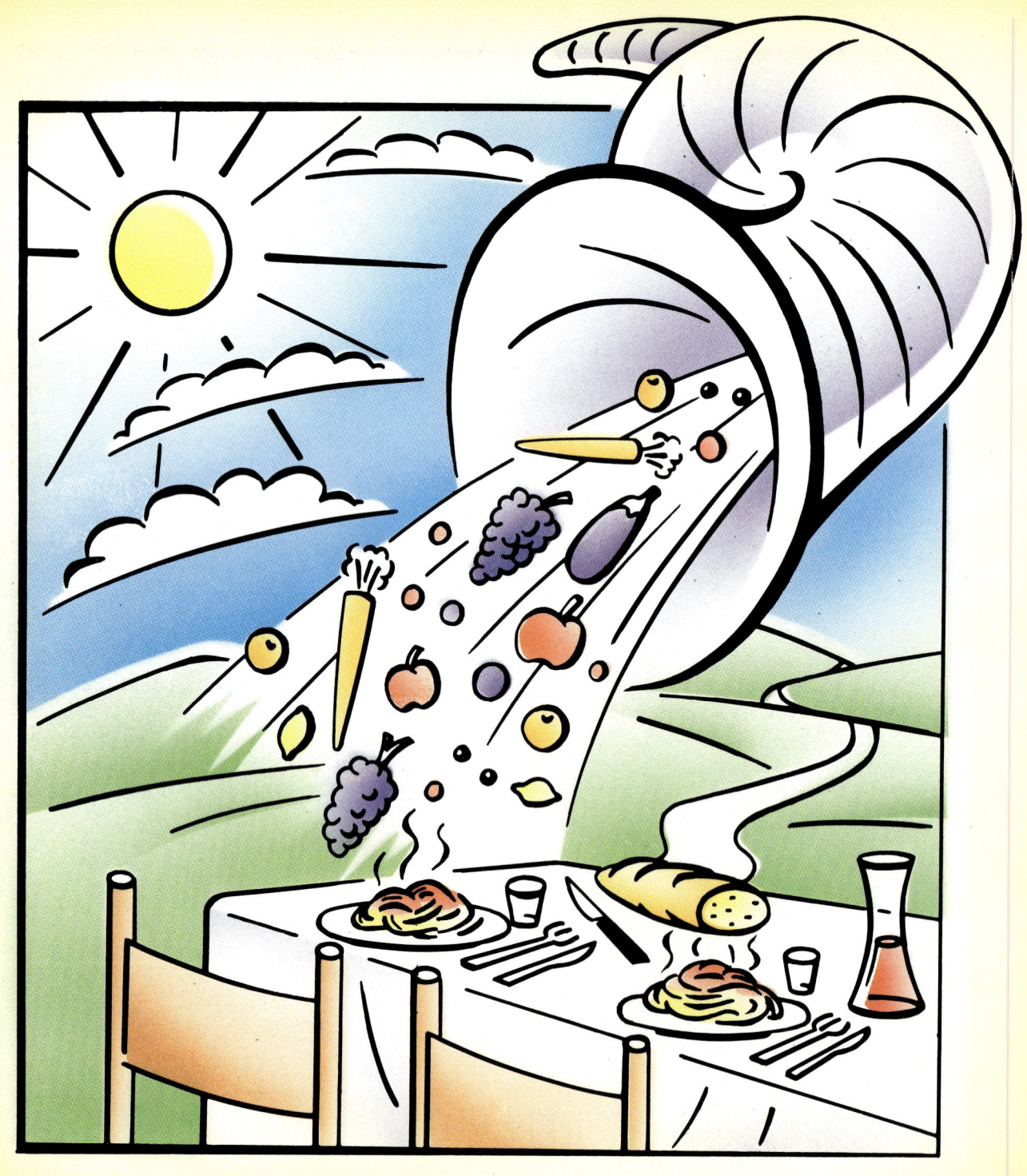

CHAPTER 5

Diet and Diabetes

By Melba Mensch, Dietitian
Diabetes Education Centre, Royal Newcastle Hospital
and
Dianne van Netten, Dietitian
Diabetes Education Centre, Royal Newcastle Hospital

To help control your blood glucose level and weight, choose, a healthy diet and get regular exercise. If you are overweight, losing weight should have a high priority in the treatment of your diabetes. Being overweight can worsen your diabetes.

Are you within the healthy weight range (*see chart*)?

Energy (joule, calorie) needs change throughout your life; therefore, your food intake will require adjustment every few years. Children, adolescents and pregnant women need extra attention.

Which foods are the right foods

The major nutrients which you will need for good health are carbohydrate, protein, fat, vitamins, minerals, fibre and water.

To control your diabetes and provide adequate nutrition your meals should be
– high in carbohydrate
– high in fibre
– low in fat
– low in sugar

Carbohydrates in your diet

Plant source foods such as bread, cereals, rice, fruits and vegetables are the major source of carbohydrates in your diet; milk providing a smaller portion. Carbohydrate source foods should provide at least half of your energy requirements. It is the carbohydrate foods which affect your blood glucose level. The sugar and starches in these foods break down to glucose which then enters your blood stream. Sugars and starches are the major source of glucose.

There are two main groups of carbohydrates – sugars and starches.

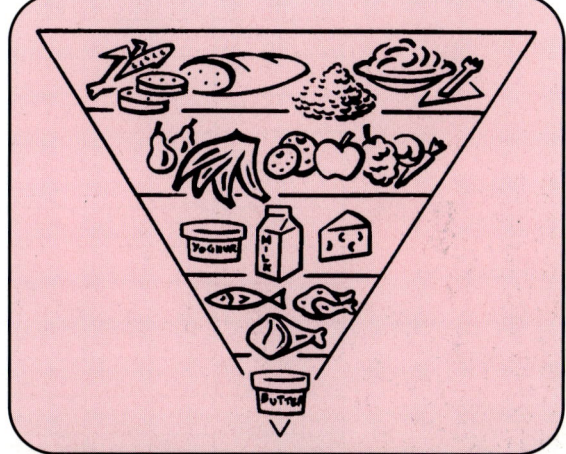

The healthy diet triangle – showing the recommended proportions of different foods.

1. Sugars –
Glucose is the sugar in our blood.
Sucrose (table sugar) is the most commonly used sugar but there are other naturally occurring sugars.
Fructose is the naturally occurring sugar in fruit. Lactose is the natural occurring sugar in milk. Fruit and milk should be included in your diet each day but too much may adversely affect your blood glucose level and weight. Fruit is best eaten raw rather than as juice because the fibre, feeling of satisfaction and some of the vitamins and minerals may be removed when juicing the fruit.
Honey is a natural sugar made by bees. Glucose is the simplest form of sugar and is added to many medicines and confectionery.

2. Starches –
Starch is the form in which plants store their energy. It is composed of a large number of

Diet & Diabetes

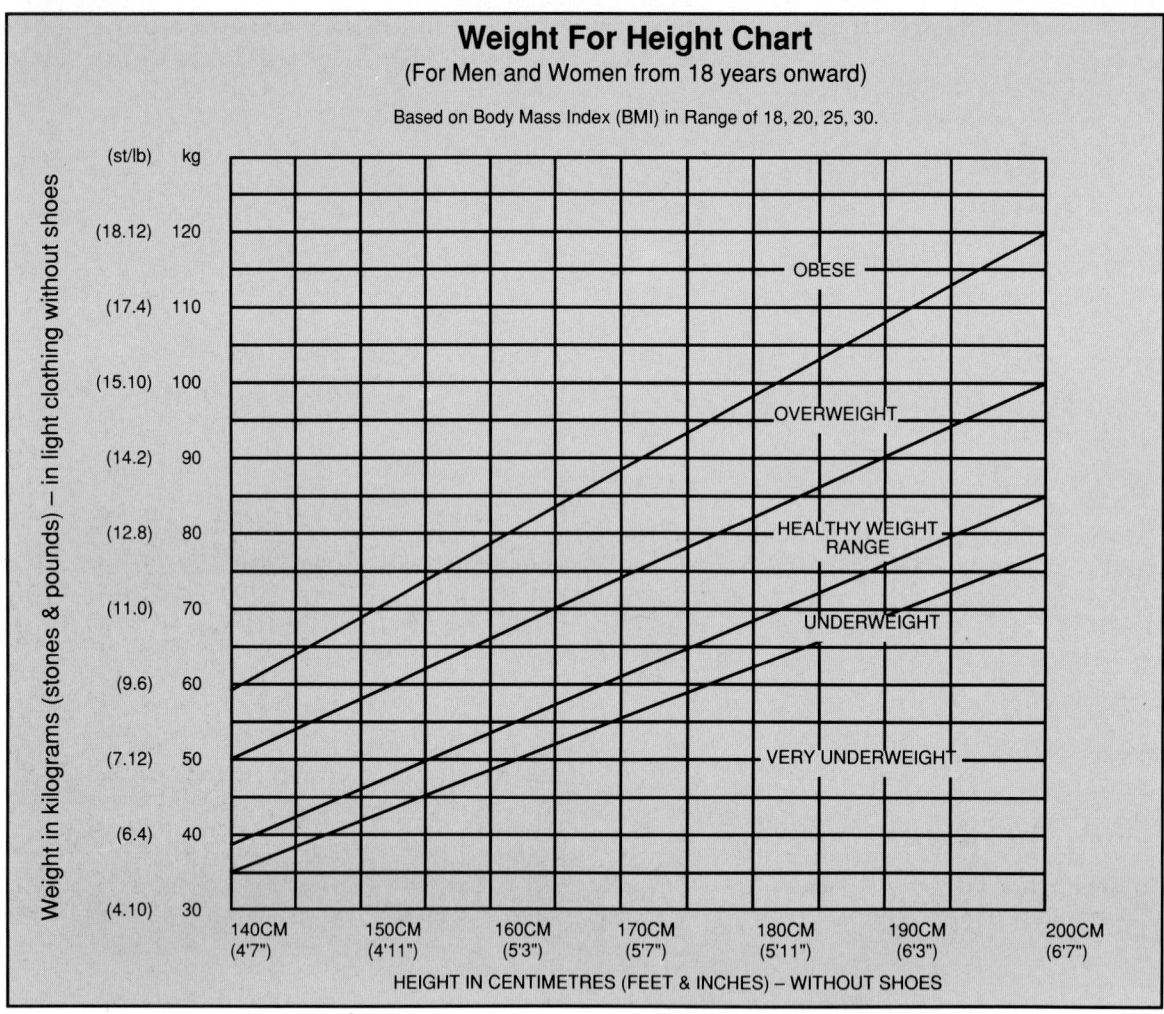

glucose units linked together. Through cooking and digestion, the complex starch molecules are broken down into glucose.

Starches are found in grains such as wheat, oats, and rye, bread, vegetables, rice, seed, llentils and dried peas and beans.

Fibre

Adding fibre to your diet has become the panacea of the 1970's and 80's. adding unprocessed bran to your diet will not make up for a fibre poor diet.

There are two types of fibre found in plants.
1. Water insoluble fibre.

These are the bran type fibres found in wholegrain products such as wholemeal bread or brown rice. Your body is unable to digest bran fibre; therefore, it is energy free. Bran fibre helps to move food around the intestines, produce a soft stool and eliminate waste products. However, bran fibre does not have an effect on the rate at which carbohydrate is converted to glucose. Foods high in insoluble fibres are wheatbran, wholegrain cereals, breads and fruits and vegetables.
2. Water soluble fibre

These types of fibres are less well known. They include fibres such as guar, pectin and agar.

Diet & Diabetes

Guar like fibres are found in legumes. Pectin is found in fruit. Agar is found in seaweed. Porridge also contains a guar type of fibre. **These fibres form a gel when mixed with the stomach contents. It is believed that the gel forms a coating around the molecules of carbohydrate. This gel makes it more difficult for the enzymes to digest carbohydrates. Therefore, the conversion of carbohydrate to glucose is slowed down.**

Choosing high fibre foods

Choose fibre rich foods whenever possible. Foods listed below are all high in fibre.
- wholemeal and wholegrain products: breads, plain biscuits, breakfast cereals, pasta and brown rice.
- pulses: legumes, lentils, dried peas and beans: all types
- all vegetables: preferably with skins
- fruit: with skins where possible – rather than fruit juice

Note on vegetables
- You can eat vegetables that are NOT starchy as freely as you wish as they are low in energy.
- Vegetables contain vitamins, minerals and fibre and can be eaten raw or cooked or included in other dishes such as soups and casseroles.

Carbohydrate Servings

To help you balance your intake of carbohydrate foods, a list of carbohydrate containing foods has been developed. Each food on each list contains the same amount of carbohydrate if consumed in the stated amount. For example 1 slice of bread contains 15 grams of carbohydrate which is equal to ½ cup potato or 1 medium apple or 2 wheatmeal biscuits.

The list has been developed to help you add variety to your meals and have a daily consistent carbohydrate intake.

Carbohydrate spacing

You may find it easier to achieve better blood glucose control if you distribute your intake of carbohydrate source foods throughout the day into 5 or 6 small meals. Include at least one carbohydrate source food at each snack and preferably two or more at your main meals. For additional information about your diet see your doctor or dietitian.

Blood glucose response (Glycaemic Index)

A slice of bread, ½ cup baked beans, ¼ cup uncooked porridge, 1 medium apple all contain the same amount of carbohydrate, therefore, you could assume that no matter which carbohydrate food you eat (in the given amount) the resulting amount of glucose entering your blood stream would be the same. However, the time taken for that amount of glucose to reach your bloodstream is different for each carbohydrate food. Look at the following example. Half a cup of baked beans has the same amount of

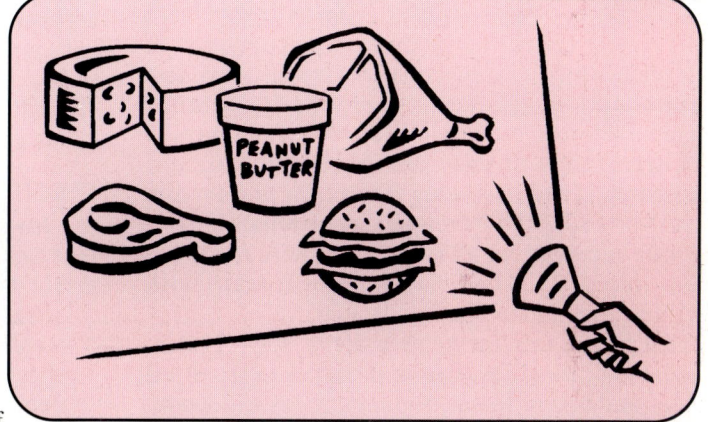

Look for visible and invisible fats – fats may be hiding in your food.

carbohydrate as ½ cup potato. However, the carbohydrate in the baked beans is converted to glucose at a slower rate than the carbohydrate in the potato.

Glycaemic Index is a system which ranks foods according to the rate at which the carbohydrate reaches your bloodstream in the form of glucose.

The glucose in foods containing water soluble fibre are the slowest to reach your bloodstream. The prime examples are: legumes (kidney beans, soya beans, baked beans, lentils, split peas) and oats.

There is a very wide range of Glycaemic Indices for all the different carbohydrate foods.

Diet and Diabetes

This makes it difficult to classify them into groups. Also, there are many influences on Glycaemic Index, for example:
– preparation methods
– processing methods, canned, frozen, fresh
– other ingredients in the food
– differences in different people for the same food

Based on what can be observed from the results of research into Glycaemic Index the following broad guidelines can be given.
– Eat legumes (dried beans, peas, lentils) and oats more often
– Choose foods containing fibre, ie vegetables, fruit and whole grain products
– avoid foods with a high sugar and/or fat content

Proteins

Every cell in your body is partly composed of protein which is subject to continuous wear and replacement. Since your body cannot manufacture protein you need to include protein source foods in your diet each day. Current research is demonstrating that a high protein diet may promote the development of renal disease. Large serves of high fat animal protein foods are not necessary. These foods often contain both visible and hidden fats.

Choose low fat protein foods such as lean meats, skinless chicken and turkey, fish, dried peas and beans, lentils, legumes, seeds and lowfat cheese, milk and yoghurts.

Fats

Fats including all types of margarines, oils, butter, cream have the highest energy content of all foods. Fat is essential but only in small amounts. Use as little as possible. Since fat is also found in many foods such as meats, cheese, eggs, you do not need to add extra fat to your food.

The fat in food is normally a mixture of 3 basic types of fat with different foods containing them in varying proportions. The energy content of all types of fats is the same.

Saturated Fats

These are of animal origin and are solid at room temperature. Saturated fats tend to raise cholesterol levels when eaten in excessive amounts.

Monosaturated Fats

Olive, canola and peanut oils, olives, nuts and avocado pears are very good sources of monosaturated fats. Monosaturated fats are beneficial to your cholesterol and other blood fat levels.

Polyunsaturated Fats

Polyunsaturated fats are usually liquid at room temperature and are extracted from plant seeds such as safflower, sunflower, corn, soya bean. Fish are also a good source of polyunsaturated oil.

Polyunsaturated fats tend to assist in lowering your cholesterol level. They also form the foundations for substances in the body called prostaglandins, some of which may protect against thrombosis (blood clotting). Fish are a very good source of three fatty acids used in the production of prostaglandins. Including fish in your diet frequently is preferable to taking fish oil supplements.

Hints for reducing fat in your diet

Invisible fats – Some foods contain fats that you cannot see. In many foods you may not be aware of its presence.

Watch out for the following:
– meats, processed and luncheon meats, sausage
– cheese, whole milk and yoghurt
– nuts, seeds, olives
– cakes, pastries, biscuits, ice cream, chocolate
– many snack foods – potato crisps, Twisties, corn chips, Cheezels
– many takeaway foods
– many gravies and sauces

Visible fats – In some foods the fat is visible and when possible avoid or remove:
– butter, margarine, oils, lard, dripping, cream, peanut butter
– fats on meat (including bacon), skin on poultry
– salad dressings, mayonnaise

Low fat options
– grill, dry roast or steam meats
– use lean meats, veal, breast of chicken, or fish often
– steam, boil or dry fry vegetables
– select low fat biscuits

Diet & Diabetes

- use low joule (calorie) salad dressings
- use skim and fat reduced dairy products including cheeses such as cottage cheese
- top vegetables and meat with low fat cheeses or vegetable sauces
- prepare meat sauces, casseroles, soups ahead of time then refrigerate and remove fat before adding vegetables or thickening

The golden rule is to use as little fat as possible when preparing or cooking food and to choose low-fat alternatives whenever you can.

Alcohol and diabetes

Alcohol can interfere with your diabetic control. It is important that you do not drink when your diabetes is in poor control. Alcohol can cause "hypos" if taken without food. Since alcohol contains joules (29 kilojoules or 7 calories per gram) people who are overweight are recommended to abstain from drinking alcoholic beverages. Excessive alcohol intake will cause damage to your liver, pancreas, brain and heart. Some basic guidelines

1. Avoid drinking alcohol on a daily basis.
2. Limit yourself to two drinks at one time.
3. Select only dry wines, spirits or beer. Avoid sweet wines and liqueurs.
4. Use low joule cordials and carbonated beverages, soda water and unsweetened mineral water as mixers.
5. Eat some carbohydrate foods while drinking alcohol to avoid "hypos" (1 portion per 2–3 drinks is sufficient).

Surviving in the supermarket

There are thousands of food items on the grocery store shelves to choose from but you may find selecting the best foods a real dilemma.

Here are a few steps that may make grocery shopping more enjoyable.

1. Read the list of ingredients. The food in the greatest amount is listed first and so on.
2. Look for added sugars. Remember there are a number of different types of sweetening agents that add energy as sugar does. Look for: sucrose (cane or table sugar), brown sugar, raw sugar, fructose, lactose, maltose, dextrose, glucose, honey, sorbitol, mannitol, and corn syrup solids.
3. If the information is available on the label check the percent of sugar that has been added to the food. If there is a choice select the food with the lower amount of sugar.
4. If none of the above sweetening agents have been added ask yourself "What has the product been sweetened with?" With new food labeling laws a code number will be used instead of the name of the artificial sweetener.

Non-energy yielding sweeteners:

Name	code number
Acesulphame K	950

Aspartame
  Equal™
  Nutrasweet™
	951

Cyclamate	952
Saccharin	954

Reduced energy sweeteners:

Sorbitol	420
Mannitol	421
Isomalt	953
Hydrogenated glucose syrup	965
Xylitol	967
Polydextrose	1200

5. There are many low joule products that are very low in energy and can be added freely to your diet. These include:
   - Low joule carbonated beverages
   - Low joule cordials and jelly
   - Low joule Gravox
   - Tablet or liquid artificial sweeteners
   - Low joule salad dressings
   - Low joule chutneys and tomato sauces
6. Some products have non-nutritive sweeteners added but contain natural sugars such as artificially sweetened peaches. These products are not energy free.

Be sure to check the labels on all new foods that you add to your shopping trolley.

Dining Out

Here are a few hints that you may find helpful when you dine out at your favourite restaurants or clubs.

Diet & Diabetes

1. Select restaurants with menus that offer a good variety of low fat foods. Some speciality restaurants may offer a very limited menu.
2. Select restaurants that are not renowned for long delays in serving meals. When making the reservation you may wish to inform the restaurant that one of your party members has diabetes.
3. If you want to dine at the restaurant later than you usually have dinner at home. Take your insulin with you to the restaurant and give your injection when your main course arrives. If you give your injection before you leave home and there is a long delay in receiving your meal you may have a hypo or you will need to eat a lot of bread.
4. Select from the menu carefully. If unsure about ingredients or cooking methods, ask.
5. Avoid foods with descriptions such as sautéd, fried, crispy, butter sauce, pan-fried, creamed, escalloped, au lait and basted.

Menu Suggestions

Entree selections – consomme soups, seafood cocktails with the sauce on the side so you can choose how much you want to use, smoked salmon, oysters naturelle, salad, cooked vegetables or fresh fruit.

Main course selections – grilled fish, lean grilled meats, baked meats, roast chicken, chinese dishes without a high sugar content such as braised chicken and chinese vegetables. When selecting pasta dishes the entree sized serve may be more in keeping within your meal plan than the main course serving. Select tomato based sauces versus the cream or cheese sauces. If you are invited to a restaurant that serves unfamiliar foods go to a bookshop or library and review recipes of some of the foods you may be served. There are many different ethnic foods on the market – why not try a few new ones?

Vegetables and salad selections – Avoid vegetables and salads to which sauces and dressings have been added. Steamed or boiled have the lowest energy value.

Dessert selections – Many desserts have a very high sugar content and in many situations a high fat content and are best avoided. Fresh fruit is an excellent choice. For special occasions ice cream may be selected.

Suitable selections can be made at "Fast food family restaurants" and takeaway bars. For food analysis of these foods ask your doctor or dietitian.

Food choice list

To help you balance your carbohydrate intake with your insulin or oral hypoglycaemic tablets and your exercise, your doctor or dietitian will assist you in developing a meal plan. The list of foods above may help you add variety to your diet.

BREAKFAST
- breakfast cereal – preferably whole-grain such as porridge, wheat flakes, or processed bran cereal, plain unsweetened muesli – with low-fat milk.
- fruit
- bread or toast – preferably wholemeal or wholegrain – with thinly spread margarine or butter (if desired).
- tea, coffee, or water.

LIGHT MEAL
- soup (if desired, preferably homemade).
- bread, roll or biscuit – preferably wholemeal or wholegrain – with thinly spread margarine or butter (if desired).
- starchy vegetables, rice, pasta, or pulses.
- salad vegetables.
- a small serve of lean meat, skinless chicken or turkey, fish, egg or low-fat cheese.
- fruit.
- tea, coffee or water.

MAIN MEAL
- soup (if desired, preferably homemade).
- starchy vegetables, rice, pasta or pulses.
- other vegetables (include freely).
- a small serve of lean meat, skinless chicken or turkey, fish, egg or low-fat cheese.
- bread or roll – preferably wholemeal or whole grain – with thinly spread margarine or butter (if desired).
- fruit or low-fat milk dessert.
- tea, coffee or water.

CHAPTER 6

The Use of Tablets

By the late Dr Pincus Taft
Former Consultant Endocrinologist
Alfred & St Vincents Hospitals
Melbourne, Vic.

Tablets have been available for the treatment of diabetes for over 30 years.

There was a drop in popularity due to concerns over safety in the 1970's but with better understanding of their actions, potential dangers and side effects, tablets - or oral hypoglycaemic agents, now have a recognised place in diabetes treatment.

Since a major part of the effect of tablets is stimulation of insulin production, they can be used only by people whose pancreas is still producing some insulin. Because of this, they cannot be used in the treatment of Type 1 (Insulin-dependent) diabetes and are confined to people with Type 2 diabetes, usually aged over 50 and overweight at diagnosis.

Tablets no substitute for diet

It is very important to note that use of tablets is restricted to situations where diet can't restore blood and urine glucose to normal levels or where diet required to lower blood glucose causes weight to fall below normal for age, sex and height.

Tablets cannot be used as a substitute to diet.

Effectiveness of tablets

Because tablets promote natural insulin production and because insulin action in Type 2 diabetes usually declines over time, it is often necessary to increase dosage of tablets to maintain ideal diabetes control.

Indeed, tablets may become ineffective in the regulation of blood sugar after a long period but good diet plays a major role - often prolonging effectiveness of tablets for many years.

Effectiveness of tablets is assessed the same way as all diabetes treatments. Of course the aim of the treatment is to relieve the person with diabetes of all symptoms and restore blood glucose levels to normal or as close to normal as possible.

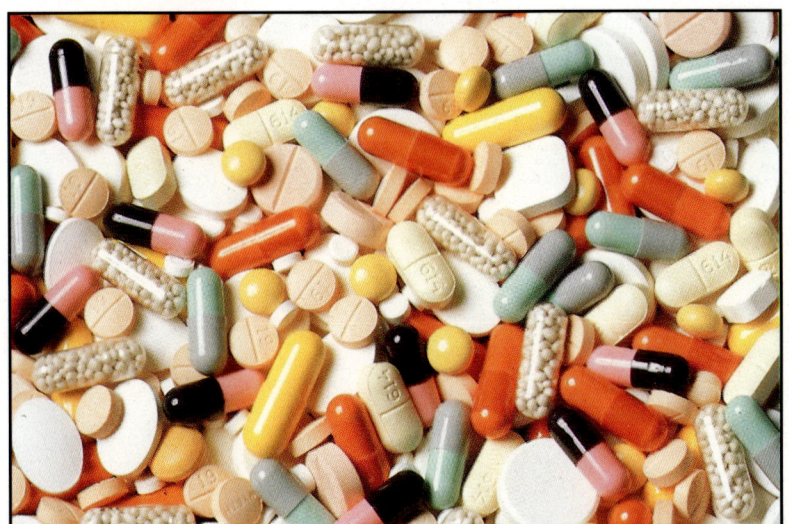

Whether this is being done will be confirmed by blood or urine glucose tests or a combination of both. The responsibility for these tests rests with the person with diabetes, and are explained elsewhere in this book (chapters 9 and 10, Self Monitoring of Blood Glucose and Testing Urine). The doctor will also carry out similar or additional tests from time to time.

The Use of Tablets

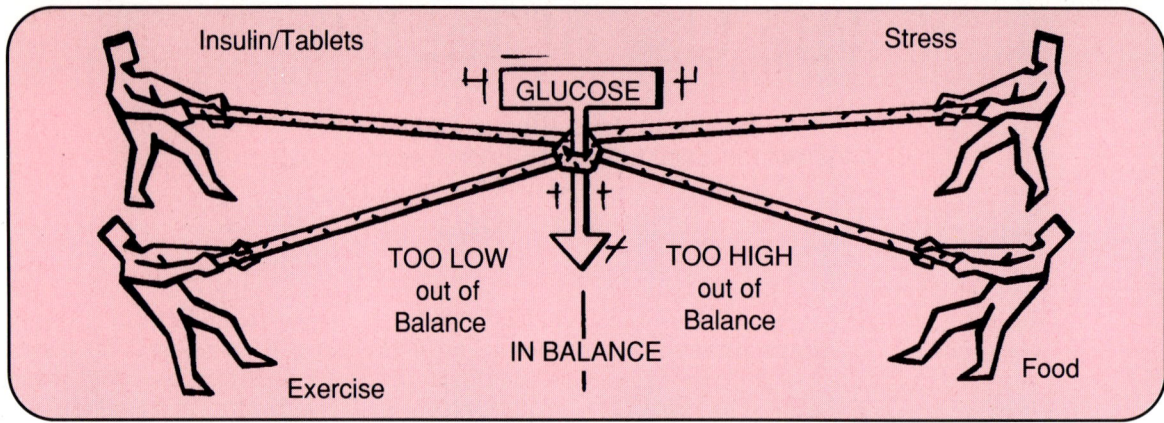

The person's weight will also be watched carefully since being underweight or overweight may call for a modification of diet or tablet treatment.

Should control be unsatisfactory or not be improved by attention to diet or adjustment of tablet type or dose, it may be necessary to transfer to insulin.

Choice of tablet and side effects

Tablets belong to two chemical "families" – the more widely used *sulphonylureas* and the less common *metformin*.

There are a number of tablets to choose from the sulphonylurea family. They vary in dosage, potency and frequency of use. Side effects can occur occasionally and include skin rashes, gastric and bowel upsets and, on rare occasions, jaundice.

Sulphonylureas can cause hypoglycaemia, just the same as insulin, where doses larger than necessary are prescribed or where food is omitted.

The second group contains only one medication, metformin, which is thought to act in a different manner. It can be used alone or in combination with a sulphonylurea.

The only significant side effects are nausea and diarrhoea (especially if the dosage is increased quickly), and these occur more commonly than with the other drugs. They are however less likely to cause hypoglycaemia and some authorities suggest they can assist diet induced weight loss.

With all these tablets, careful assessment of the user's health is made to ensure safety. Heart, liver and kidney disease may make them unsuitable for use. If they do not work satisfactorily, their use will be stopped and insulin substituted.

Remember that other medication may affect diabetes medication and control (chapter 14, Diabetes and Other Medications).

The use of tablets when ill

Just as with people who have a successful control with diet and insulin, illness such as 'flu or gastroenteritis can upset the use of tablets.

Such intercurrent illnesses can cause increased blood and urine glucose levels with a recurrence of symptoms of diabetes – thirst, urinary frequency and vomiting.

Just as much attention must be given to people with diabetes using tablets as using insulin and they should seek medical treatment if intercurrent illness effects control. In such a case additional treatment with insulin may be needed.

This is also true in the case of pregnancy where, if diet does not achieve control, insulin is the preferred treatment.

The Use of Tablets

ORAL HYPOGLYCAEMIC AGENTS AVAILABLE

Chemical Name	Brand Name	Tablet Size	Daily Dose Range	Approximate Duration	Frequency (Times/d)	Administration	Potency	Side Effects
Chlorpropamide (a)	Diabinese	250mg	125-500mg	36h	Once	With Meals	Strong	Hypoglycaemia, Weight gain, Jaundice, Alcohol Flushing, Low sodium levels, Skin rashes, Blood disorders
Gliclazide (a)	Diamicron	80mg	40-320mg	18-24h	1-2	With Meals	Intermediate	Hypoglycaemia, Weight gain, Skin Rashes, Blood dyscrasis
Glibenclamide (a)	Daonil, Euglucon, Glimel	5mg	2.5-20mg	18-24h	1-2	With Meals	Strong	Hypoglycaemia, Weight gain, Skin rashes, Blood disorders
Glipizide (a)	Minidiab	5mg	2.5-40mg	6-12h	1-2	With Meals	Strong	Hypoglycaemia, Weight gain, Skin rashes, Blood disorders
Metformin (b) (c)	Diabex, Diaformin, Glucophage	0.5g	0.5-3.0g	12h	2-3	With/After	Weak	Hypoglycaemia is rare, Anorexia, Vomiting, Diarrhoea, Lactic Acidosis
Tolbutamide (a) (d)	Rastinon	0.5 & 1.0g	0.5-3.0g	8-12h	2-3	With Meals	Weak	Hypoglycaemia, Weight gain, Skin rashes, Blood disorders

Note: Oral agents should be used with special care in the elderly.
(a) Sulphonylurea (b) Biguanide (c) Care renal, liver and cardio-vascular disease (d) Choice in renal disease

DIABETES & YOU
An owner's manual

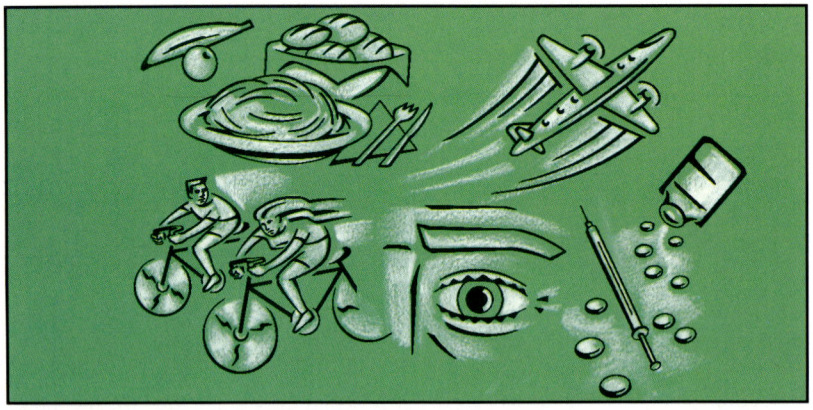

INSULIN AND MONITORING

❏ **Types of Insulin**

    Uses of different insulins
    Strengths
    Storage
    The right dose
    Adjusting the dose
    Problems you may encounter
    Injection devices
    Infusion systems

❏ **Injections and Injectors**

    Choice of syringe
    Choice of needles
    Withdrawing insulin
    Choosing a site
    Giving the injection
    Possible side effects
    Automatic injectors
    Jet injectors
    Children and injections

❏ **Self Monitoring of Blood Glucose**

    Reasons for monitoring
    Frequency of testing
    Testing schedules
    Factors influencing blood glucose tests
    How to test
    Care of strips
    Buying a meter
    Obtaining a drop of blood
    Safe disposal of used lancets

❏ **Testing Urine**

    Renal Threshold
    Testing for glucose
    Testing for ketones
    Testing for proteins
    When to test
    Recording results

❏ **Hypoglycaemia and Hyperglycaemia**

    Symptoms
    The most common causes
    Treatment

❏ **Diabetes and Exercise**

    What happens during exercise
    How to manage diabetes during exercise
    Advice on insulin or tablets
    Other important considerations
    What types of exercise
    How much exercise

❏ **Sick Days**

    Monitoring blood and urine
    Insulin or tablets
    Extra insulin
    Food and drink
    Vomiting
    In hospital

❏ **Diabetes and Other Medications**

    Medications that may raise blood glucose
    Medications that may lower blood glucose
    Medications that alter response to glucose or insulin
    Medications which can affect urine glucose tests
    Unusual interactions
    Interactions with complications of diabetes

CHAPTER 7

Insulin and Its Role

By Dr Frank Alford
Director, Endocrinology Unit
St Vincents Hospital
Melbourne Vic.

For some people with diabetes, daily injections of insulin are part of their life – as much a matter of routine as eating breakfast or brushing their teeth. But what is insulin, and why is it so important if you have diabetes?

Well, insulin is a hormone which enables energy giving blood glucose to enter body cells such as muscles. This movement of glucose out of the bloodstream and into the cells lowers blood glucose levels. Normally a perfect balance between glucose entering the blood and glucose leaving it will be created.

In the case of diabetes, the pancreas does not make enough insulin and this perfect balance and the normal blood glucose level it creates, cannot be achieved naturally. The body needs help and, as insulin cannot be given in tablet form, this means daily insulin injections either by syringe or pen devices.

There are many different forms of insulin, made by various manufacturers, bearing various brand names and possessing different features. Despite that, there are only three sources of insulin: human – made in the laboratory, beef extracted chemically from beef cattle and porcine – extracted chemically from pigs (porcine insulin is now only available in Australia under special circumstances).

Each is available in either short acting insulin with effects which last six to eight hours; medium, up to 24 hours; and long acting, which can last up to 36 hours.

All insulins available do basically the same job. They all lower blood glucose levels. One unit of short acting insulin will have the same capacity to lower blood glucose as one unit of long acting. The difference is the amount of time it takes to do it.

The choice of which type of insulin is best suited to the person's particular needs and lifestyle will be made by the doctor and patient together.

This choice – and the education process which goes with it, is most important. The person with diabetes must know which insulin they use and what its properties are. It is not advisable to switch randomly from one insulin to another, despite how similar their names and qualities might seem.

The dosage is vital. Too much insulin will result in too great a fall in blood glucose. This leads to what is called a hypoglycaemic attack commonly known as an insulin reaction or "hypo".

By the same token, not enough insulin will fail to lower the blood glucose level enough, resulting in persistently high blood glucose and poorly controlled diabetes.

With that in mind, there are a number of points to remember:

- *Type of insulin used and the daily dosage.*
- *Time of the insulin's maximum effect and duration of action.*
  This is important because the time of maximum effect, the time when the insulin is at its greatest strength and working hardest, is the time the person with diabetes is most likely to have a "hypo" reaction.
- *Regular timing of injections and meals.*
  Eating regular meals at regular times is necessary to balance the effect of the insulin. It may also be necessary to take snacks between meals on advice of your doctor.
- *Report to the doctor any change in lifestyle, working hours, physical activity or meal times*
  All these factors, along with stress, can affect the control of diabetes.

Insulin and Its Role

TABLE A
TYPES OF INSULIN COMMONLY USED
TIME OF ACTION IN HOURS AFTER INJECTION

TYPE OF INSULIN		OVERALL EFFECT	START OF EFFECT Hours	MAXIMUM EFFECT (Greatest Chance of Hypoglycaemic Reaction – Hours)	END OF EFFECT Hours	APPEARANCE	SPECIES OF INSULIN
Generic Name	Trade Name (at Feb 1994)						
Insulin Acid	Insulin 2	Short acting	1-2	3-6	7-8	Clear	Beef
Neutral (Soluble)	Actrapid / Humulin R / Hypurin Neutral	Short acting	½-1	2-4	6-8	Clear	Human / Human / Beef
Isophane (NPH)	Humulin NPH / Hypurin Isophane / Isotard MC / Protaphane	Intermediate acting	2	4-10	16-18	Cloudy	Human / Beef / Beef / Human
Insulin Zinc Suspension (Lente)	Humulin L / Lente MC / Monotard	Intermediate acting	2	6-12	16-24	Cloudy	Human / Beef / Human
Isophane plus Neutral Mixed Insulin	Humulin* / Mixtard**	Mixed Short & Intermediate acting	1-2	2-12	16-18	Cloudy	Human / Human
Insulin Zinc Suspension (crystalline)	Humulin UL / Ultratard / Ultralente MC	Long acting	2-6 / 2-6	6-20 / 6-20	24 / 36	Cloudy	Human / Human / Beef
Protamine Zinc Insulin (PZI)	Protamine Zinc Insulin MC	Long acting	4-6	14-24	36	Cloudy	Beef

* Available in various mixtures of neutral and isophane 20:80, 30:70, 50:50.
** Available in various mixtures of neutral and isophane 15:85, 30:70, 50:50.
NOTE: *As there is a difference between human and animal insulins, discuss fully with your doctor any proposed transfer between human and animal insulins.*

Insulin and Its Role

The most important thing though is to <u>ASK QUESTIONS</u>. It is vital to have access to all information on diabetes and its treatment. If there is anything you are not sure about, ask your doctor and insist on answers you can understand.

Types of insulin

As we have said, the treatment of diabetes is very much an educational process, learning about the condition and the ways to control it. An initial discussion with a doctor about diabetes and the various types of insulin will probably seem confusing.

Don't panic. No-one can be expected to grasp all that information at one sitting. Once you have started to become more familiar with insulin, you will be able to go back to your doctor and discuss it further. Then, feeling more confident and in control, together you will be able to determine the best way to make treatment of your condition fit in with your lifestyle.

The tables on pages 26 and 30 give you examples of widely used types of insulin and how they work in relation to your day. You will see that they all have different brand names but don't let this worry you. The actual type of insulin – or generic name, always appears on the label, so as long as you know the type of insulin you need, the brand name should not confuse you.

Basically though, there are four types of insulin: Short-acting, Intermediate acting, Mixed (Short and Intermediate), and Long-acting.

Short-acting insulins, which are also known as soluble or neutral insulins, have their maximum effect from about three to six hours after injection, with the effects wearing off rapidly after about eight hours. They are clear in appearance.

Intermediate-acting insulins are cloudy and have their maximum effect between eight and fifteen hours after injection. This means they will be working hardest in the mid afternoon or early evening after a morning injection, thus the need for a mid afternoon snack to balance the insulin action.

Mixed Short and Intermediate Acting insulins contain mixtures of the two in various amounts. For instance a mixture of three parts short-acting to seven parts intermediate is available as are various other combinations.

Long-acting insulins last up to 36 hours.

Uses of different insulins

Short acting insulins are most commonly used when control is needed quickly or when some complicated situation has arisen, such as acute infection or surgery.

They can also be used in standard day to day treatment, either several times a day on their own – usually with a pen device rather than syringe, or fewer times per day in combination with intermediate or long acting insulins.

Intermediate acting insulins are usually used in standard day to day control either once or twice daily.

Long acting insulins have become more popular recently because they can be used with short acting insulins which are given with pen-devices. However they can bring on a reaction during the night with some people.

Human vs beef vs porcine

There is a slight difference in the structure of beef, porcine and human insulins but each works very effectively. With the correct dosage, each will effectively control diabetes. Human insulin is manufactured whereas beef and porcine insulin are obtained from the pancreases of cattle or pigs. Porcine insulin is only available in special circumstances.

Because they differ in their time of maximum effect and length of action, it is not recommended to switch between the insulins from different sources. If it is necessary to change from one to the other, this should only be done under the close supervision of a doctor.

Strength of insulins

All insulin preparations carry a label to indicate their strength, on the basis of how many units of insulin there are in one millilitre (ml) of the solution. In Australia, this is 100 units per ml, signified on the label as U 100.

U 100 insulin has taken over in Australia from U 40 and U 80, but in some countries these

Insulin and Its Role

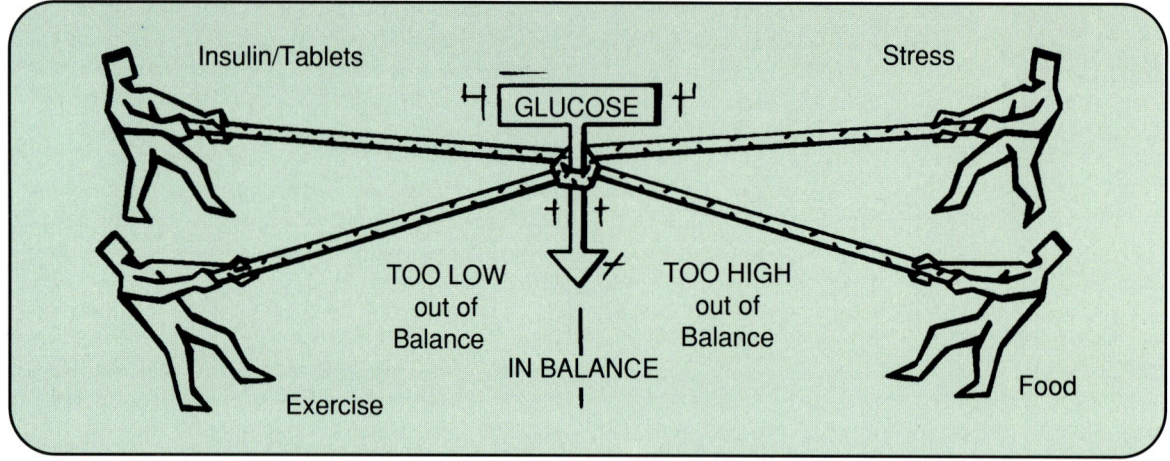

strengths are still common. This means, when travelling overseas extra care must be taken to check the strength of the insulin. U 40 or U 80 insulin should not be used with the standard Australian U 100 syringe or the dose will be wrong. (See chapter 27, Travel).

To be sure though, no matter where you are, you should always check that the chemist and doctor have given you the correct type of insulin, and always check the **expiry date** on the label.

Storage of insulin

The bottle of insulin you are using can be kept in a cool spot in a room. Bottles not in use should be stored, on their side, in a refrigerator not the freezer.

Insulin is destroyed by heat and so must not be left in the car glove box or elsewhere where temperatures may exceed 40°C.

Finding the right dose

In most cases, help is available to find the right dose of insulin. This is because treatment usually begins in a hospital or diabetic treatment centre, as an outpatient.

There you will be taught a number of things, such as injection techniques, storage of syringes and needles, interpretation of blood and urine tests and how to recognise and treat a reaction.

At this time, working together with hospital staff and your doctor, a dose will be worked out for you. This is fine in principle, but your needs may be different away from the controlled environment of the hospital. It will only be when you are back home, going about your usual activities that the proper dose can be ascertained and once again, this is something you must work out in close contact with your doctor.

Adjusting the dose

Some people are reluctant to change their daily dose of insulin without consulting a doctor or nurse, but there are situations in which it may be necessary to do so.

For instance, there could be a change of diet or increase in activity at work. You may have a minor infection or be under stress.

All these things will mean your usual insulin dose does not have the level of control it should. In such cases, it is desirable to adjust the dose to keep the blood glucose at a satisfactory level – but at the same time, it is important not to change the dosage too much and risk an insulin reaction.

To do this, you will need confidence and experience, but a general rule is that it is quite safe to vary your insulin by up to one tenth of your regular dose. That is, two units if you are taking up to 20 units per dose, four units if you are taking 20 to 40 units per dose and six to eight units for a dose of between 40 and 80 units.

Through your own experience, and by keeping a careful daily record, you will know whether larger variations can be made safely.

Generally speaking, an increase in insulin

Insulin and Its Role

will be necessary to counter a mild infection, inactivity, increase in food and some instances of extreme stress.

A decrease will be necessary after recovering from infection, with increased activity or when food intake is likely to be less than normal. Dosage should also be decreased if insulin reactions have been occurring for no apparent reason.

The menstrual cycle may also affect diabetic control, and it is not unusual for women to need different doses of insulin before, during and after periods.

Ideally, the insulin dose should be tailored to match regular test results, as measurement of blood glucose levels is the best guide to proper control. This is why it is so important to record the results of your regular blood level tests. If you have this information, you can use it to make the right decision at the right time.

Many people with diabetes test their own blood glucose levels using blood glucose meters between one and five times a day or every second day. A common practice is to measure blood glucose levels before each meal and before bed. Sometimes people may check in the middle of the night if they feel themselves becoming "hypo".

A guide to interpreting blood glucose levels is in chapter 9, Self Monitoring.

Control charts for varying insulin dosage are available and your doctor or nurse can explain how to use them. There are however some basic rules which you should follow:

- *Know your condition* – have a good working knowledge of your diabetes.
- *Know your insulin* – remember its time of peak action and total duration.
- *Test regularly* – and monitor results.
- *Record test results* – and use your records to make informed decisions.
- *Consider your diet* – often a change of diet can be as useful as a change in insulin dosage.
- *If in doubt, ask your doctor or diabetes nurse.*

Problems you may encounter

There are some problems associated with using insulin, but most are rarely encountered and usually temporary.

One which can be avoided through knowledge and practice, is faulty injection technique. If insulin is injected into the skin instead of under it, it may cause a painful local reaction, with redness around the injection site.

The correct technique is explained in Chapter 8, Injections and Injectors.

Reaction brought on by faulty technique occurs immediately after injection. This is different from another rare problem, local allergy, which occurs an hour or two afterwards.

This type of reaction, which consists of a painful reddened area and itching, usually occurs on the first couple of months of using insulin, and goes away after one or two months.

The problems of loss of fatty tissue or hollows (fat atrophy) and the formation of fatty tissue or lumps (fat hypertrophy) are both rare today because of the use of purified insulins. These problems are usually avoided by rotating the site of injection each day.

There are also two types of systemic – or generalised, immune reactions, both of which are very rare.

They either come in the form of a skin rash with or without swelling or, as insulin resistance which is generally taken to mean a daily requirement of more than 200 units of insulin.

Injection devices

Over the past few years, a number of new devices – such as the "insulin pen" have been introduced to help the diabetic with the regular injection of insulin.

These devices are described fully in Chapter 8, Injections and Injectors, but simple and convenient as they are, they do not lessen the need for a full understanding of insulin and how it works, or the need for diligent blood glucose monitoring.

Insulin infusion systems

A recent development has been the mechanical infusion pump which uses short acting insulin, delivered at a low rate at night and between meals, and at a high rate at meal times.

❏ ❏ ❏

Insulin and Its Role

TIME-ACTION OF VARIOUS INSULINS

TYPES OF INSULIN			
Generic Name	**Trade Name**		**ACTION**
Insulin Acid	Insulin 2		
Insulin Neutral (Soluble)	Actrapid * Humulin R** Hypurin Neutral		SHORT ACTING
Isophane (NPH)	Humulin NPH** Hypurin Isophane Isotard MC Protaphane *		INTERMEDIATE ACTING
Insulin Zinc Suspension (Lente)	Humulin L Lente MC Monotard		
Biphasic-mixed Isophane plus Neutral Insulin	Humulin** 20/80, 30/70, 50/50 Mixtard 15/85, 30/70, 50/50		MIXED SHORT AND INTERMEDIATE ACTING
Insulin Zinc Suspension (Crystalline)	Humulin UL Ultralente MC Ultratard		LONG ACTING
Protamine Zinc Insulin (PZI)	Protamine Zinc Insulin MC		

FOOD INTAKE

B S L   D   S   B
7 12   7   12   7
am mid pm   mn   am

B breakfast   D dinner
L lunch   S snack
              Z sleep

FOOT NOTES

The trade names given here are those in use at February 1994. Additional trade names will be introduced from time to time but the generic name always appears on the label, so you can compare the generic name with this table.
* Also available in Penfills.
** Also available in Cartridges.

Insulin and Its Role

Insulin is a silent partner. It is the agent which controls the balance in the blood, and it will do its job for you, effectively, efficiently and without drama as long as you do your part.

That is – remember the type, dose and labelling code of your insulin, remember the time when it has its peak effect and its duration of action. Remember to take your insulin and meals regularly each day.

And just as importantly, remember when in doubt, ask your doctor or diabetes nurse.

CHAPTER 8

Injections and Injectors

By Associate Professor Alan Stocks
Visiting Physician
Dept of Diabetes and Endocrinology
Princess Alexandra Hospital
Brisbane

The type of diabetes which requires treatment with insulin injections usually occurs in children and young adults. Soon after diagnosis the correct technique required to give an injection and the dose needed will be explained by the doctor or diabetes nurse.

This will happen either in hospital or at a diabetes clinic, but when the person with diabetes goes home and gets on with day to day life, daily injections will become a matter of routine.

The doctor or diabetes nurse will always be there if you get into difficulties, but the everyday management of your diabetes ultimately rests with you. Therefore, it is vital that injections are given correctly and insulin measured accurately.

As explained earlier, insulin cannot be absorbed through the stomach and so there is no alternative but to inject it. This can be done with syringes, pen injectors or even a special infusion system. They can all do the job.

Now obviously no-one enjoys having injections, but it can be made a lot less uncomfortable by using the right equipment and the correct technique.

Choice of syringe

The syringe must be marked clearly with a suitable scale. As explained, there is only one strength of insulin available in Australia (U-100) and standard syringes are available from state branches of Diabetes Australia or from chemists or some hospital diabetic clinics.

The most commonly used syringe has a total capacity of 1 ml, marked with 50 lines along its side – one every two units. The major divisions, 10, 20 ,30 etc, are marked with a number and longer line.

A smaller syringe with a total capacity of 1/2 ml- usually used for children, and a rarely used 2ml syringe are also available. The 1/2 ml syringe is marked with 50 divisions—one for every unit of insulin. Major divisions every five units are marked with a number and a longer line.

Both are available in either glass or disposable plastic.

The disposable plastic syringes are the simplest to use and are especially useful when sterilisation is a problem. They are designed to be used once only but many people use them safely for eight to ten injections if the needle is neither blunt nor bent. The syringe must be recapped and kept dry in a cool place between injections, although it is not necessary to keep it in the refrigerator. Disposable syringes should not be resterilised in methylated spirits.

Choice of needles

Most disposable insulin syringes have fixed needles. For glass syringes, a 26, 27 or 28 gauge needle 12.5 or 15.1 mm in length should be used to draw up and inject the insulin – it is not necessary to use the larger "drawing up" needle to withdraw insulin from the bottle.

Withdrawing insulin from the bottle

All techniques for treating your diabetes will be discussed and demonstrated by your doctor or diabetes nurse soon after diagnosis but the recognised routine for withdrawing insulin from a bottle is:

1) Wash and dry hands.
2) Gently swirl the bottle or turn it upside down to mix and suspend the insulin (but do not shake the bottle.) This is especially important with cloudy insulins which should become an

Injections and Injectors

even suspension. Ultralente insulin usually only party suspends and it is not necessary to make it completely smooth before drawing it into the syringe.

Bottles with obvious particles which stick to the inside of the bottle should be thrown out.

Clear insulin should be just that – clear, and bottles with sediment floating in them should also be thrown out.

3) If a glass syringe is being used, assemble the syringe and needles, being careful not to touch the needle tip. Pump the syringe with air to push out anything which might be inside it.

4) Withdraw the plunger to measure the same amount of air as the required dose of insulin.

5) Invert the insulin bottle. Holding it firmly, pierce the centre of the cap with the needle and inject air into the bottle. Draw the plunger down again and insulin will then flow easily into the syringe to replace the amount of air injected.

Note that it is not necessary to swab the top of the insulin bottle before use.

6) Tap the syringe barrel gently with one finger to send any air bubbles up into the bottle. This is sometimes difficult with plastic syringes, but if only a few tiny bubbles remain this will not matter.

7) When the bubbles are expelled, adjust the plunger to measure the exact dose of insulin.

8) Withdraw the needle from the bottle. The syringe now contains the correct dose.

9) Inject the insulin.

Withdrawing a mixed dose

If you need to withdraw insulin from two bottles for a mixed dose:

Follow steps 1, 2 and 3 above, then

4) withdraw the plunger on the syringe to measure the same amount of air as the required dose of cloudy insulin. Inject this air into the cloudy insulin bottle but do not withdraw the insulin. Instead, with the plunger fully pressed

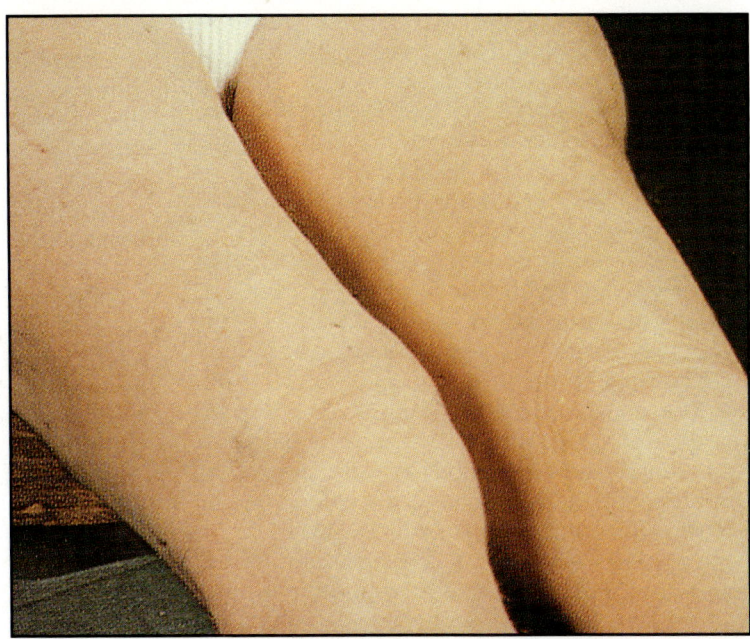

Fatty lumps caused by repeated injections into the same area.

down, remove the needle from the bottle. This leaves the positive air pressure inside the bottle.

5) Measure air in the syringe to equal the required dose of clear insulin.

6) Inject this air into the clear insulin bottle.

7) Withdraw the required amount of clear insulin and expel the bubbles.

8) Reinsert the needle into the cloudy insulin bottle and carefully pull down the plunger to withdraw the required cloudy insulin.

If you accidentally withdraw too much cloudy insulin, do not press the plunger to return it to the bottle, as this will put clear insulin into the cloudy bottle. Simply remove the bottle, expel all insulin from the syringe, and start again from step 4.

9) Inject the mixture.

When drawing up mixed doses always draw up the two insulins in the correct order.

Choosing the site of the injection

The best places for injections are those where a loose fold of skin can be pinched up. These are the abdomen, upper outer thighs, buttocks, or upper outer part of the arm.

For girls and young women it is not advisable to inject insulin into the arms as the development of lumps or hollows may be cosmetically

Injections and Injectors

undesirable. It is best to use unexposed areas on the abdomen, buttocks and upper thighs.

The injection should be given in a different place each day as repeated injections in the same place may cause tissue changes that will delay the absorption of the insulin or make it unpredictable. Eventually a tough, fatty lump may form.

Therefore it is necessary to vary the site, but in a calculated systematic way. If, for example, the abdomen is used, the site should be varied by about two cms each day, moving along imaginary lines running up and down.

The injections can be given as far as the rib margin and down to the level of the pubic hair and around to the side as far as you can see. The only area on the abdomen which should not be used is one inch (2.5cm) around the navel.

It should be possible to place eight to ten injections on each line and fit in at least 10 lines two cms apart across the abdomen. Imagining the abdomen squared off like a grid, it should be possible to fit in up to 100 injections before using the starting spot again.

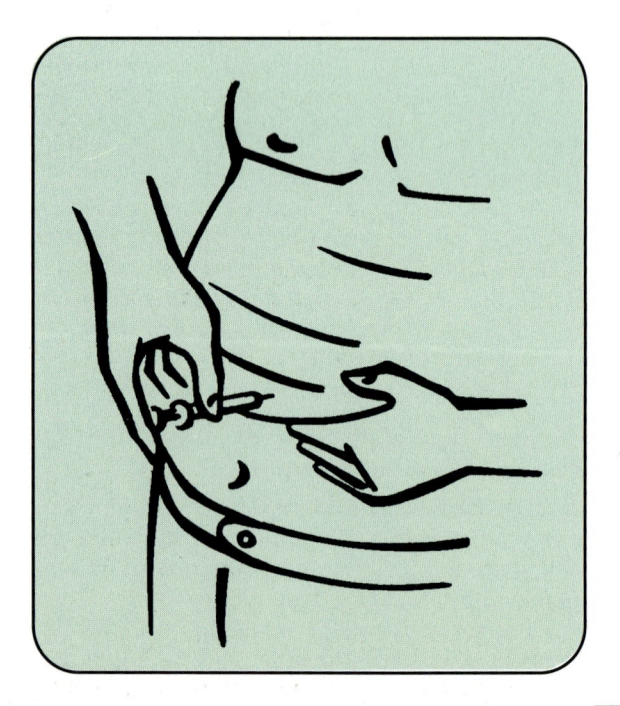

Where not to inject

Insulin should never be injected into the inner side of the arms or the inner side of the thighs or groin creases because that is where large nerves and blood vessels are near the surface.

Areas which show networks of fine veins are best avoided to reduce the risk of bruising.

Giving the injection

Once again, the technique of giving an injection will be well discussed and demonstrated by the doctor or diabetes nurse. There are two standard routines.

A 1) If the injection site is dirty, it should be cleaned with soap and water. It is not necessary to swab the area with spirit as this increases the likelihood of a painful injection.

2) Grip the syringe like a pencil between the fingers.

3) With the other hand pinch up a mound of the cleansed skin, 2-3 cm across.

Hold the syringe at an angle of about 60 degrees to the skin- that is, not pointing directly inwards but at a slight angle off vertical. If using the right hand to inject into the right thigh, point the syringe slightly downwards towards the knee. If using the right hand to inject the left thigh, it will be easier to point the syringe slightly upwards toward the hip.

4) Insert the needle to the full length at an angle of 60 degrees.

5) Let go the pinch and grasp the bottom of the syringe. This releases the other hand to operate the plunger.

6) Gently raise the plunger to check that the needle is not lying in a blood vessel. If blood appears in the syringe when the plunger is raised withdraw the needle and start all over again.

NOTE: Only a very gentle upward pressure is needed. If the plunger does not withdraw very easily, it is most unlikely that the needle tip lies in a blood vessel.

7) If no blood appears in the syringe, inject the insulin slowly.

8) Withdraw the needle and press firmly over the injection site. Do not rub the site. If bleeding

or bruising occurs, press firmly for two or three minutes.

B) An alternative simpler method is to hold the syringe between the thumb and middle finger leaving the index finger free to push the plunger.

Pinch up an area of your abdomen (preferably) with your other hand.

Insert the needle at slight angle off the vertical. Slowly push in the plunger to inject the insulin dose. Withdraw the needle, release the pinched up area.

If a disposable needle or syringe is used, it should be disposed of safely. It should be placed in a metal or a stout plastic container. Contact your local council or Diabetes Australia concerning arrangements for disposal.

If a glass syringe is used, pump the syringe 10 times with the needle still attached to remove the surplus insulin, then return the syringe to its container. If the syringe is sterilised in spirit, it is not necessary to rinse with boiled water.

Local Skin Reactions

There are several kinds of local skin reactions, including:

STINGING which may occur at the site of injection when insulin is cold, when injecting through alcohol from a swab or when treatment is first started. This kind of reaction is most common with soluble insulin, which is acid. A change to neutral insulin such as Actrapid, Humulin R or Velosulin may solve the problem, but the doctor should be advised as soon as it occurs.

MILD LOCAL ALLERGY which may cause tender itchy red lumps at the injection site usually occurs during the first few weeks of treatment with beef insulin but is extremely rare with human or porcine insulin. It may be caused by the injection being too shallow, so make sure the insulin is being injected deeply enough.

Usually this problem solves itself after a few weeks and it is not necessary to change the type of insulin being used.

HOLLOWS (fatty atrophy) – the wasting of fatty tissues under the skin, is a problem rarely encountered since the introduction of highly purified insulins. It is more common among women than men, more common when long acting insulins are used, and much more common when insulin is injected cold. As mentioned earlier, insulin should always be injected at room temperature to prevent hollows forming. If an area is rested from injections for several weeks, the hollows will sometimes disappear.

LUMPS (fatty hypertrophy) – a lump or swelling, is particularly common in children. Repeated injections into a small area produce a fatty lump at the injection site. Therefore, injection sites must be changed frequently, as the

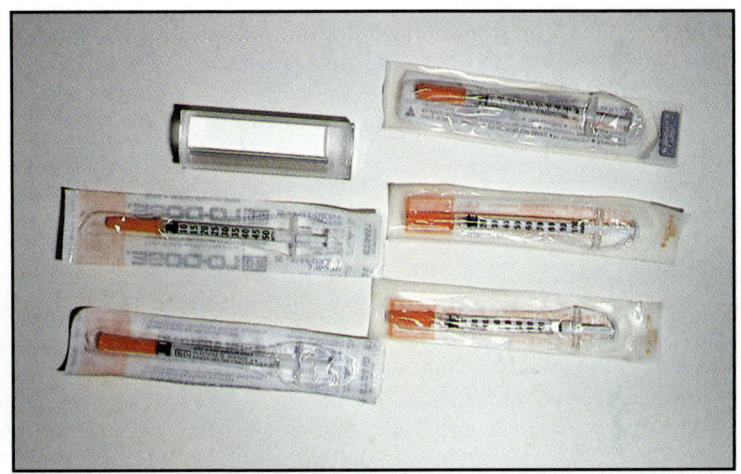

All the syringes currently available are accurate, reliable and cause minimal discomfort.

absorption of insulin from fatty lumps is unpredictable and leads to poor diabetic control. Also, if the area of injection is changed after the lump has formed, the more rapid absorption of insulin from the new site may cause an unexpected "hypo". Lumps usually disappear slowly over several months when insulin is no longer injected at that site.

BRUISING will occur occasionally, no matter where the insulin is injected. One preventative is to avoid obvious networks of veins and keeping movement of hands and syringe whilst injecting to a minimum.

General Reactions

GENERAL ALLERGY to insulin affecting

Injections and Injectors

the whole system is very rare but if it should occur it may produce a skin rash, fever and joint pains. Such symptoms should be reported to your doctor immediately.

INSULIN RESISTANCE, due to the antibodies in the system which reject insulin. This is very rare since the introduction of highly purified insulins.

Using pen injectors

As already stated there are a number of pen devices available on the Australian market.

The NovoPen I looks like a fountain pen but when the cap is unscrewed and fitted on to the other end of the pen, a small plunger appears and it becomes a syringe. Disposable insulin cartridges containing 150 units of Novo insulin such as Actrapid HM, Protaphane HM and Actraphane HM fit into the NovoPen.

Pressing the plunger down completely delivers two units of insulin, and a double click is easily heard. Pushing the plunger down halfway delivers a single click, and one unit of insulin.

As the cartridge empties, a red rubber bung can be seen moving down through a window on the side of the pen. When it reaches a white line on the cartridge, there are ten units remaining.

When replacing the cartridge, it is important to hold the NovoPen vertically with the needle downwards so that the ratchet device inside the lid falls into the new cartridge and comes to lie hard against the rubber bung, or else depressing the plunger may not deliver insulin.

The NovoPen II is larger and fatter than the NovoPen I but uses the same cartridges and needles. The insulin dose is preset by twisting the end section of the pen anti-clockwise and a distinct click is heard for each two units of insulin added. A locking ring is then twisted, after which the insulin can be injected by pressing a plunger at the end of the pen.

The locking ring is a safety device, but can be very stiff and hard to use by people with a weak grip.

When the NovoPen II is used with cloudy insulin it is important to ensure the mixture is evenly suspended by rolling the pen between the hands and inverting it several times before use.

SITE CHOICE: The rate of absorption of insulin varies with each site. The best area is the abdomen. Other sites eg. buttocks, thighs, could be used. The injection should be given in a slightly different area each time. This will help the insulin absorption and avoid "fatty" unsightly lumps.

The Insuject Pen is designed to use Nordisk's Velosulin Insuject cartridges which contain 250 units of human insulin. The cap unscrews anti-clockwise, revealing the needle and needle guard. The dose of insulin can be preset by twisting the grooved sleeve at the other end of the pen.

A click is heard as each unit is added, so that the pen may be used safely by blind or partially sighted people. The insulin is injected by twisting the grooved sleeve back to the zero mark.

When the grooved sleeve is pulled back away from the needle end, a scale is revealed which indicates the number of units left in the cartridge. When the scale is no longer visible, there are fewer than 10 units left.

The popularity of the Insuject Pen led to requests for a pen which could take Insulatard insulin. In response Nordisk developed the Insuject-X which differs from the Insuject pen in several ways so that there is no danger of confusing the two.

Amongst these differences, there is a window on the side of Insuject II allowing a clear view of the insulin suspension, the cap unscrews clockwise – the opposite of the Insuject and a clicking noise can be heard as the cap is unscrewed.

Injections and Injectors

Replacing the cap on the pen extracts the needle from the cartridge automatically, preventing leakage of insulin between injections. Removing the cap automatically re-inserts the needle into the cartridge and the pen is ready for use.

The method of presetting the insulin dose is the same as with the Insuject, but each click represents two units of insulin.

Once again, it is important to ensure the Insulatard insulin is evenly suspended by rolling the Insuject-X pen between the hands and inverting it several times before use.

The Humulin range of insulins is presently being used in conjunction with an insulin pen manufactured by Becton Dickinson and it is anticipated that this will soon be available in Australia.

Automatic injectors

Some people find automatic injectors to be of great benefit if they are not confident about giving themselves injections. These devices have a mechanically controlled spring which thrusts the needle through the skin quickly.

Some also depress the plunger automatically but these are not recommended because there is a risk the insulin will be injected too closely under the skin.

Devices such as the Busher injector insert the needle mechanically but the plunger has to be pushed by hand, making this device less liable to error.

There are some claims that automatic injectors provide total pain-free injections but this is hard to accept. Some require special syringes and these may not conform to the Australian Standard for insulin syringes.

Jet Injectors

A number of jet injectors such as the Preci Jet are now available and have the advantage that it is not necessary to inject a needle as the injection device fires a jet of insulin through the skin at high speed.

Such devices are extremely expensive, need frequent sterilisation by boiling in distilled water, are too bulky to be easily carried around, and drawing up the insulin is more complicated than with syringes. Injections are usually, but not always, painless and bruising at the injection site occurs just as often as with ordinary syringes and pen injectors.

Jet injectors may be useful for people with diabetes who cannot bring themselves to inject with a needle, such as young children or people with a nervous disposition, but cannot be recommended for the majority of people with diabetes.

Devices for people with poor eyesight

There are a number of devices which enable safe and accurate measurement of doses for the blind or partially sighted. The B-D Scale Magnifier clips on to an insulin bottle and ensures the needle of a standard insulin syringe will puncture the rubber cap of the bottle in the centre. It also magnifies the markings on the syringe three times.

Another device known as the Deckerject is designed for use with Terumo syringes.

The Hypoguard "click-count" syringe can be used safely by people who are totally blind. The dose of insulin can be varied and it is not necessary to preset the syringe. Mixtures of insulin can be given with a "click-count" syringe.

Pen injectors can also be used safely by people who are blind or partially sighted and who wish to continue giving their own injections.

Most States have Low Vision Clinics which can give useful advice.

At what age should children give themselves injections?

This question, often asked by parents, has no set answer. It depends when diabetes is first diagnosed. Children who have had diabetes from infancy are often very independent and comfortable with injections at a very early age.

The answer is best left to the child, however newly diagnosed children as young as six years old often have little fear of needles and may adapt more quickly to the diabetic routine if allowed to give their own injections from the beginning.

In fact, a problem might be caused if a parent

Injections and Injectors

does not give responsibility to the child early enough. It is common for resentment of injections to occur when a parent keeps giving injections until the child is aged 10 or 12.

An ideal time for a child to start giving injections is at a Diabetic Children's Camp, when children wary of giving injections have the opportunity to see others their own age taking charge of their own treatment.

Safe disposal of needles, syringes and lancets

Care should be taken at all times when handling needles, syringes and lancets. Supplies should be stored carefully and, where necessary, in a child proof cabinet.

Needles and lancets should only be recapped by the person who has had the injection or finger prick. Only containers approved by Diabetes Australia should be used to store used needles, syringes and lancets. A growing number of local councils will receive and exchange sharps containers at little or no cost.

❏ ❏ ❏

Still, the key to this and so much else remains knowledge, through which confidence and understanding can be established. Whether people with diabetes administer the injections themselves or a relative or nurse does it for them, it is the job of the doctor or diabetes nurse to ensure all information is readily available.

If there are any doubts, any problems, any fears, just ask. This is your body, your responsibility. Take charge.

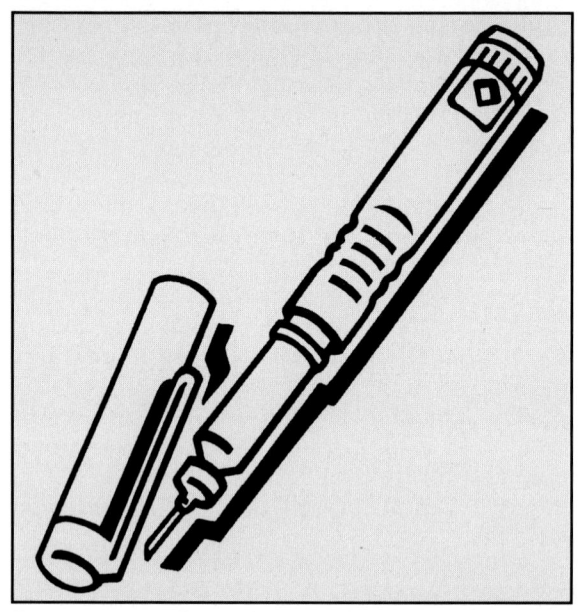

Pen injectors make insulin administration simpler and more convenient.

CHAPTER 9

Self Monitoring of Blood Glucose

By Trisha Dunning
Clinical Nurse Consultant
Diabetes Education
St Vincents Hospital
Melbourne

In order to go about their everyday life, people with diabetes must know what their body is doing. Effective control of diabetes is all about maintaining a satisfactory balance within the bloodstream and therefore it is necessary to regularly monitor blood glucose levels to know the dosage of insulin or tablets and the amount of food and exercise which will create that balance.

Monitoring blood glucose is not a complicated procedure requiring complex equipment. It is something which can be fitted into usual activities, as part of a regular routine. By providing information necessary for effective diabetes management it is a tool to help maintain quality of life and therefore should not be seen as a nuisance or means of control by health professionals.

After diagnosis, you should be taught the appropriate blood glucose monitoring technique and the reasons for testing should be fully explained. It is important that follow up advice is available should you need it.

Reasom for blood glucose monitoring

The main reasons for testing blood glucose are:
- To monitor the effectiveness of diabetes treatment and to serve as a guide for you and the doctor in planning adjustments of medication doses.
- To show the relationship between blood glucose, food, exercise and diabetes tablets/insulin.
- To define unacceptable control as indicated by blood test results.
- To diagnose hypoglycaemia including nocturnal hypoglycaemia.
- To detect unstable or "brittle" diabetes.

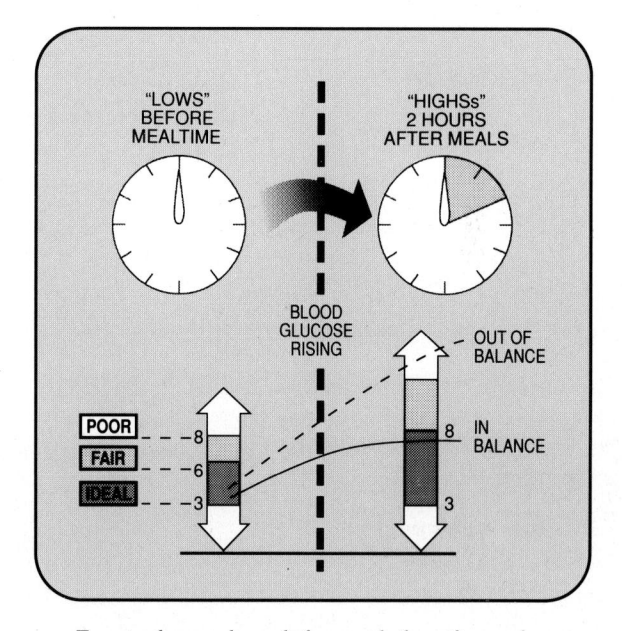

Target values are lower before meals than afterwards.

- To manage "sick days" at home, and when recovering from an illness.
- To monitor the response to a new treatment schedule such as stabilisation on to insulin.
- To provide continuity of care following admission to hospital for illness or an operation. To establish the renal threshold and the reliability of urine testing for glucose.
- To achieve ideal diabetic control during pregnancy.
- To assist people with nerve damage (neuropathy) to recognise hypoglycaemia.
- To achieve an acceptable blood glucose range, which may have a role in preventing or delaying the onset of diabetes related complications.

Self Monitoring of Blood Glucose

Frequency of testing

The number of tests and the target blood glucose range will be established in consultation with the doctor and will depend on the level of control, your age and the method of treatment.

If you have any problems which may make testing difficult (such as arthritis in the fingers and problems with your eyesight) they should be discussed with your diabetes advisers to discuss such aids as meters with enlarged numbers which can help overcome these problems.

Testing schedules

Blood glucose is usually tested before meals, and in some cases two hours after eating.
Some common schedules are:-
- Three or four tests each day, if diabetes is unstable or if treatment is being altered, and usually in young people with type 1 diabetes.
- Daily or twice daily tests, changing the time of day at which the test is done, if the diabetes is stable.
- One or two tests each week, if diabetes is stable, especially for those on diet control.

During periods of illness it may be necessary to test more frequently.

Blood glucose range

In Australia the units used to measure blood glucose are called millimoles (one rounded teaspoon of sugar has the equivalent of 30mmol of glucose). The following table is a guide to blood glucose levels:

Risk of hypo	less than 3mmol/L
Normal	3 – 8mmol/L
Ideal control	3 – 6mmol/L before meals up to 8mmol/L after meals
Fair control	6 – 8mmol/L before meals 8 – 11mmol/L after meals
Poor control	8mmol/L or more before meals 11mmol/L or more after meals

During pregnancy levels of 3-8mmol are required to reduce the risks of complications for both the mother and baby.

In elderly people a range of 5-15mmol may be acceptable, provided there is no thirst, frequency or tiredness causing discomfort.

Very tight control (tests in the low range) increases the risk of hypoglycaemia.

Factors which can influence blood glucose tests

There are several outside influences which can affect the results of tests.
These include:
- FOOD – time of last meal, quantity and type of carbohydrate and fibre.
- EXERCISE – timing with regard to food, medication and insulin injection site.
- MEDICATIONS used for diabetes control oral agents, insulin.
- ILLNESS – such as flu.
- OTHER MEDICATIONS – such as oral contraceptives or steroids which may be needed to treat other illnesses.
- ALCOHOL – amount consumed and its relationship to food intake.
- STRESS – both emotional and physical and medications used to treat stress may mask perception, especially of hypoglycaemia.
- TECHNIQUE – the accuracy of the monitoring technique, including not handwashing before testing if sweet substances such as jam have been handled.
- PREGNANCY – in people with diabetes and gestational diabetes.
- CHILDHOOD – erratic swings in blood glucose are usual.
- ADOLESCENCE – hormonal factors during adolescence can affect results.
- DISEASE – such as kidney, liver and pancreatic disease, and other endocrine disorders such as thyroid disease.

How to test

The technique for testing blood glucose levels involves putting a drop of blood from a fingerprick on to a special strip impregnated with enzymes which react with the glucose in the blood.

Blood is wiped, washed or blotted from the strip after a set time which allows a colour change to occur. The strip may be read by comparing its colour to a colour chart, or automatically in a blood glucose meter.

Results are recorded in a record book which

Self Monitoring of Blood Glucose

should be taken to the doctor each visit.

It is important to remember that if technique is not accurate, or tests are not timed precisely, the results will not be correct. Also, only certain strips can be used with blood glucose meters.

The key points to remember about testing are:
1. Get a good drop of blood
2. Time accurately
3. Remove blood correctly
4. Check meter regularly

The most common strips available in Australia

ACCUTREND GLUCOSE

For use in the Accutrend meter. Visual comparison is limited.

BETACHEK (National Diagnostic Products)

A drop of blood is placed on the strip and left for 30 seconds. Blood is wiped off the strip using a soft tissue. The colour is allowed to develop for a further 60 seconds (total 90 seconds) then compared with colour blocks on the container.

BM-TEST-GLYCEMIE 20/800 (Boehringer Mannheim)

A drop of blood is placed on the strip and left for 60 seconds. It is wiped at exactly 60 seconds using cotton wool. Colour is allowed to develop for a further 60 seconds then compared with colour blocks on the side of the container. If the reading is 17mmol/L or more it should be compared again 60 seconds later.

EXACTECH STRIPS

These strips can only be used with the ExacTech blood glucose sensor. Visual comparison is not possible.

GLUCOFILM (Bayer Diagnostics)

A drop of blood is placed on the strip and left for 40 seconds. Blood is removed by pulling the Glucofilm strip through a tissue. The colour is allowed to develop for an additional 20 seconds (total 60 seconds) then compared with the colour blocks on the container. Glucofilm can also be used with the Glucometer 3 and Glucometer M+ meters.

GLUCOSTIX (Bayer Diagnostics)

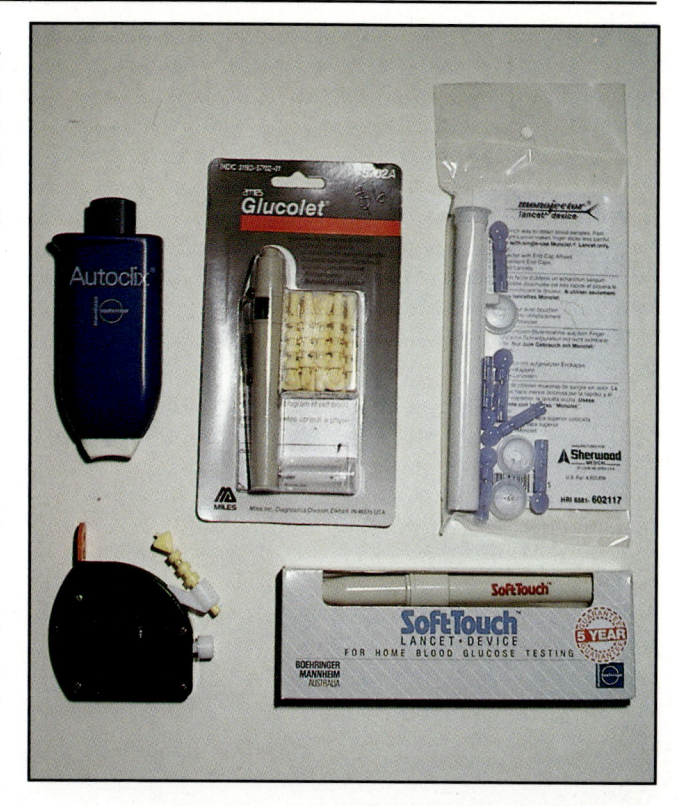

A drop of blood is placed on the strip and left for 30 seconds. It is blotted at exactly 30 seconds using a soft tissue. Colour is allowed to develop for a further 90 seconds (total 120 seconds) then compared with the colour blocks on the container.

HYPOGUARD G.A. (Astral Scientific)

A drop of blood is placed on the strip and left for exactly 30 seconds. The strip is blotted at 30 seconds. Colour is allowed to develop for a further 60 seconds and compared with the colour blocks on the back of the container.

A small plastic device has been designed to be used with the Hypoguard GA strip to assist in applying blood and to wipe the blood off automatically, as the strip is removed.

All these strips have acceptable accuracy over a wide range of blood glucose values, provided the timing is accurate and they are used in accordance with the manufacturer's directions.

The colour of the BM-Test-glycaemie strips

is stable for 2-3 days. The colour fades more quickly from both Glucostix and Hypoguard strips. Stability of colour can be useful if you are uncertain of how to interpret results and wish to check your readings with your doctor or diabetes nurse. The date and the time of the test should be recorded on the strip.

Blurred vision and disturbances of colour vision may make interpretation of the colour difficult. Any such difficulties should be discussed with the doctor or diabetes nurse.

Care of strips

Strips can be damaged if exposed to heat, light or moisture. It is important to keep the container tightly capped with the packet of chemicals (the desiccant) inside. Store at room temperature.

The expiry date which is stamped on each container should be checked before use. It is not recommended that strips be cut in half to save money.

Meters available in Australia

Before deciding to purchase a meter it is wise to examine those available to determine which one is best suited to your needs. Always make sure you are fully instructed on how to use the meter.

The <u>ExacTech Blood Glucose Meter</u>, supplied in Australia by Farmatalia Carlo Erba, uses an electrolytic method to measure blood glucose. The meters come in a fountain pen size which is small, light and easy to carry, and a credit card size with a larger display window. The ExacTech meters deliver a reading in 30 seconds and must be used with ExacTech strips. The strips are individually wrapped in foil and are available on the NHS and NDSS schemes. Strips cannot be visually read.

This meter is simple to use and gives rapid results.

Each pack of strips contains a calibrating strip and the meters should be calibrated for each pack. High and low solutions are available to check the accuracy of the meter.

The batteries are non replaceable and have a life span of approximately two years, or 2000 tests.

The <u>Ames Glucometer</u> is supplied by Bayer. The latest model, the Glucometer GX is a small lightweight meter with a large display window. It is only available in kit form, containing audio cassette, strips, control solution, fingerprick device and lancets, carry pack and the meter.

The meter should be calibrated for each bottle of strips using the on/off button. The meter has a memory recall system.

It can only be used with Ames Glucostix reagent strips.

The batteries are non replaceable and last for 5,000 tests – or approximately five years. There is a five year warranty.

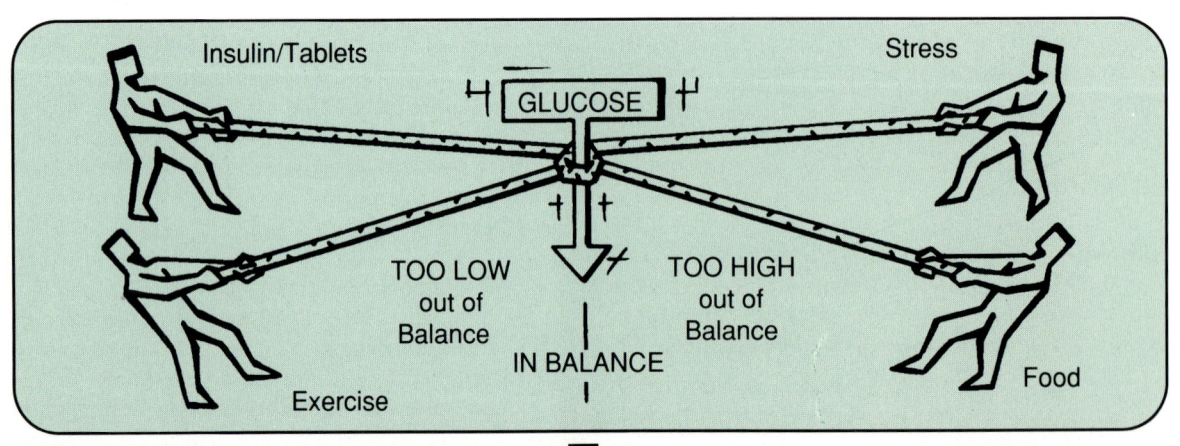

The <u>Reflolux</u> is supplied by Boehringer Mannheim. The latest model, the System S is also a small lightweight meter and uses the BM 20/800 reagent strips. The meter is calibrated with a "bar code" strip supplied with each bottle of strips. The strips hold their colour well and can be checked by your doctor or diabetes nurse in the next 2-3 days. The test takes two minutes to complete. The meter has a memory recall system. It is battery operated and the batteries are replaceable.

<u>Hypocount GA</u> is a small meter which uses the Hypoguard GA strips. The display area is large and clear. There is a memory recall which also gives an average of past results. The batteries have a life span of 12 months or 1,000 tests.

Buying a meter

Some health funds offer a rebate on the purchase cost of meters and this should be checked with your fund before purchase. A doctor's letter is sometimes required stating that a meter is needed for monitoring diabetes. It is also important to check the availability of back up service before purchase, should repairs be necessary.

If buying meters overseas it is wise to check the cost and availability of strips in Australia, as well as the availability of back up service and the display values which may not be in mmol/l.

Quality Control

Most manufacturers provide a fluid to check that you, the strip and the meter are working correctly. The fluid acts as a control of the quality of results (hence the name). You should get values within a certain range. If your value lies outside this range something is wrong with the strip, the meter or your technique. A regular check is wise—eg once a week, once a page in your record book or each time you open a bottle of strips.

Reasons for inaccurate results

An inaccurate blood glucose reading can result in the following instances.
METERS

Using the wrong strip for the meter. Using an incorrect calibration or code. Using strip incorrectly (not being exact with the recommended times) or facing the wrong way. Insufficient blood on the strip will give a falsely low reading. Using an unclean meter (with a spot of blood on the window). Using an old, discharged battery, the meter may not display a result.

BOTH METERS AND VISUAL

Blood wiped from the strip too soon can give low readings. Blood left on the strip too long can give high readings. Too forceful wiping of the blood off the strip gives low readings. Incomplete removal of blood from the strip makes interpretation difficult.

Touching the pad of the finger onto the test strip leads to patchy colour development and difficulty in reading. Strips used after the expiry date may not be accurate.

Failure to wash hands before testing, especially if sweet substances have been handled can cause high readings.

If in doubt repeat the test.

If still in doubt have your machine tested.

How to obtain a drop of blood for glucose testing

The correct technique for carrying out an accurate blood glucose test will be explained by your doctor or educator. If in doubt, continue to ask questions until you feel comfortable with the procedure.

It is important to assemble all equipment before you commence the test. That is:
  Blood test strip and meter, if used
  Lancet (Monolet, Unilet)
  Cotton wool or tissues
  Wrist watch with a second hand
  Record book
- Wash and dry hands thoroughly.
- Squeeze blood towards the tip of the finger.
- Prick confidently with the lancet on the side of the last segment. (An automatic fingerpricking device may be used).
- Squeeze towards the end of the finger till a large drop of blood has formed. It may help to hang the hand downwards if experiencing difficulty, and to warm the hands.

Complete the test according to the system chosen. Do not use the same finger for every test, and do not prick the pads of the fingers. The ear lobes may be used, although it is difficult to apply the blood to the strip without assistance.

The feet should never be used except in the case of infants, where blood can be obtained from the heel.

Equipment should be cleaned and stored correctly after use.

Self Monitoring of Blood Glucose

POPULAR GLUCOSE METERS AVAILABLE – FEBRUARY 1994

METER SERIES	REAGENT STRIP	MEMORY FACILITY	COMMENTS
Bayer series			
GX	Glucostix	Yes, stores and averages last 10 results.	Cheaper than other meters, small size.
Glucometer 3	Glucofilm	Stores 10 values	As above.
Glucometer M+	Glucofilm	Yes. Events such as meals, insulin, exercise can also be recorded.	
Boehringer Mannheim Series			
Reflolux S	BM Test Glycemie 20-800	Yes, 20 memory spaces. Interfaces with Camit for computer analysis.	Good service backup. Will show "OFF" signal if unclean, "ERR" if insufficient blood. Easy to calibrate.
Accutrend	Accutrend Glucose	Stores time and date of 50 values.	Result in 12 seconds. No wiping of strips. Limited visual colour comparison.
Accutrend Mini	Accutrend Glucose	Last reading.	Result in 12 seconds. No wiping of strips. Compact, convenient to carry.
ExacTech series			
ExacTech Pen	ExacTech	Last reading	Needs immediate press of button for accurate result.
ExacTech Companion	ExacTech	Last reading	As above.
Medisense Pen	Medisense	Yes, 10 values stored.	Auto start, result in 20 seconds, one step calibration, small size.
Medisense Companion	Medisense	Yes, 10 values stored.	As above.
Hypoguard Series			
Talking Hypocount "B"			For visually impaired. Special strip guide available to assist accurate placement of blood on strip.
Hypoguard GA	Hypoguard GA	Yes, 10 values stored.	
Hypocount Supreme	Supreme Blood Glucose test strips.		No wiping strips, visual colour comparison of strips.

Note: This table includes only currently available meters.

Self Monitoring of Blood Glucose

Automatic fingerpricking devices available

Fingerpricks are almost painless if an automatic device is used. The most commonly used devices in Australia are:-
- BM Soft Touch
- Ames Glucolet
- BD Autolance
- Autolet II -- Astral Scientific
- Clinistik 2 – General Diabetes Services

All these devices are simple to operate, are spring loaded and durable given reasonable care. All have easy to follow operating instructions and allow an adequate drop of blood to be obtained.

The Glucolet and Soft Touch have two different sized caps, one allows deeper penetration of the lancet and is used if the fingers have very tough skin.

Most people prefer to use a device rather than the lancet alone. Lancets should be used once only and discarded.

Safe disposal of used lancets

For information on safe disposal of lancets see page 38.

❏ ❏ ❏

The regular monitoring of blood glucose levels does not have to be a hassle and can play an active part in maintaining a happy, enjoyable quality of life.

CHAPTER 10

Testing Urine

By Clin. Assoc. Professor Paul Moffitt
Royal Newcastle Hospital
Newcastle

Testing the urine can be a simple and efficient means of checking the level of glucose (often referred to as sugar) in the blood.

The kidneys form urine by taking water and unwanted substances out of the blood and then discarding them through the bladder.

The kidney, like a computer, constantly measures the concentrations of substances in the blood and when excessive amounts are present, they are passed freely into the urine. For example, if the blood is deficient in salt, the kidney will retain as much as possible in the blood. If it has too much salt, the kidney will allow as much as possible to escape into the urine.

The concentration of these substances is broadly predictable, and the person with diabetes tests for variations from the normal.

There are three substances which should not appear in the urine under normal circumstances glucose, ketones and protein.

This is where testing the urine become a useful tool in the control of diabetes. Just as a barometer helps a weatherman to predict a storm and a fuel gauge shows a motorist whether he has enough petrol, regular urine tests keep the person with diabetes informed about the state of the blood glucose.

The kidneys will usually not permit glucose to be present in the urine until the level in the blood rises above 10 mmol/L, as in Figure 1. This is known as the renal threshold for glucose "renal" meaning pertaining to the kidneys.

The renal threshold is a spill-over point. In other words, the kidney – like a dam, holds back normal amounts of glucose in the blood, but when the renal threshold is reached, glucose spills over into the urine. A person with a normal threshold who has glucose in the urine must therefore have recently had more than 10 mmol/L of glucose in the blood – as in Figure 2.

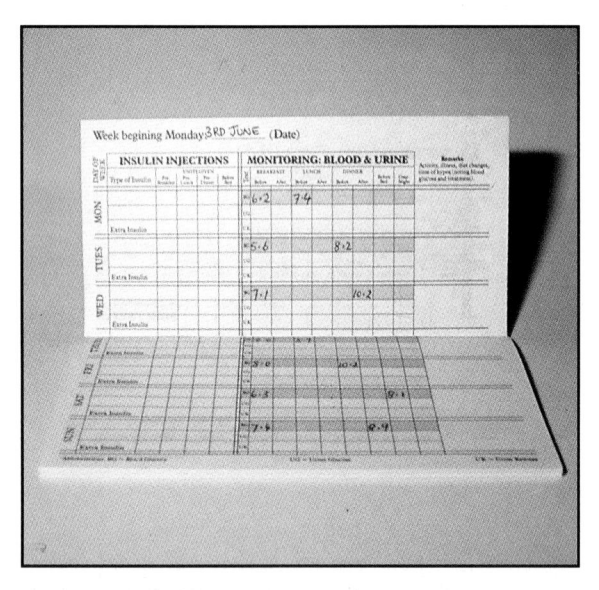

Some people may be born with or develop a low renal threshold, meaning their kidneys allow glucose to escape from the blood into the urine when the amount in the blood is actually normal. Former welterweight boxing champion of Australia Al Bourke, for example, was found to have glucose in his urine and incorrectly diagnosed as having diabetes. For the next 30 years he thought he had diabetes, and wondered why the treatment always made him feel funny. Eventually he was found to have a low renal threshold and all treatment was stopped.

Pregnant women sometimes develop a low renal threshold at around the 6 or 7 months mark and will show glucose in the urine even though blood glucose levels are normal. The threshold will return to normal after the birth.

The renal threshold can increase with age or for no apparent reason and it is therefore common for some older people with diabetes to have high levels of glucose in their blood even though their urine is completely free of glucose.

As seen in Figure 3, a low or high renal threshold will render urine testing useless as a means of assessing the level of glucose in the person's blood. The person with a low renal threshold will be tricked into believing he or she has high levels of glucose in the blood when the urine shows glucose, while the person with a high renal threshold will be deluded into believing everything is alright because there is no glucose in the urine.

Because of this it is most important that the person with diabetes and the doctor know whether the renal threshold is normal before urine testing is considered.

All methods of testing urine for glucose are based on a scale of glucose concentration but this scale cannot be used to determine the level of blood glucose. In other words, the percentage of glucose in the urine rarely equates to the level in the blood because so many factors can affect the concentration in the urine. For instance, while the presence of 2 per cent glucose in the urine does mean a high blood glucose level, the presence of only 0.5% glucose in the urine does not necessarily mean a moderate level of glucose in the blood. In fact, it could be quite high.

Testing for glucose

The most common methods of testing for glucose are:
- CLINITEST TABLETS which are used in conjunction with a Clinitest kit, consisting of a small glass tube, dropper and testing tablets. Rather impractical for use outside the home, Clinitest tablets can also falsely indicate glucose in the urine if the user is taking large doses of aspirin or vitamin C.
- DIASTIX, KETO-DIASTIX, CLINISTIX strip-testing materials are dipped quickly in and out of the urine. Small, individual sticks, easily carried in a pocket or handbag, these are convenient, for use at work or outside the home. Accurate timing with a watch is essential to get a proper reading and care must be taken not to use after the expiry date. Of these, Diastix has the best range of colour reading to show how much glucose is in the urine.
- TESTAPE is similar to strip testing, but is a tape rather than individual sticks. It is popular because the container is compact and easily carried.

All these products are available from Diabetes Australia.

Testing for Ketones

The presence of ketones in the urine – known as ketonuria, indicates that the body has switched from glucose to fat as an alternative source of energy, or food for the body cells. Its presence in the urine is not a good sign for people with Type 1 diabetes.

The presence of moderate or heavy ketones in the urine plus large concentrations of glucose is an ominous sign and the patient should contact a doctor immediately as he or she could be developing keto-acidosis (diabetic coma). If the person is also feeling sick or vomiting, the matter is urgent.

The presence of a trace of ketones in the urine of a healthy person with diabetes when they get out of bed in the morning has two possible explanations – if the urine contains only ketones and no glucose, it suggests the patient has had low blood glucose levels during the night because of too much insulin, too much exercise or not enough food the previous evening.

If the trace of ketones is accompanied by a large amount of glucose in the urine, the most likely explanation is that the person has had a deficiency of insulin during sleep.

Medical opinion differs on how often a person with diabetes should test urine for ketones. It is also essential for people with diabetes to test for ketones during any acute illness such as 'flu or other infection.

Many people use a strip which tests for both glucose and ketones and are therefore able to test for ketones several times a day.

Testing Urine

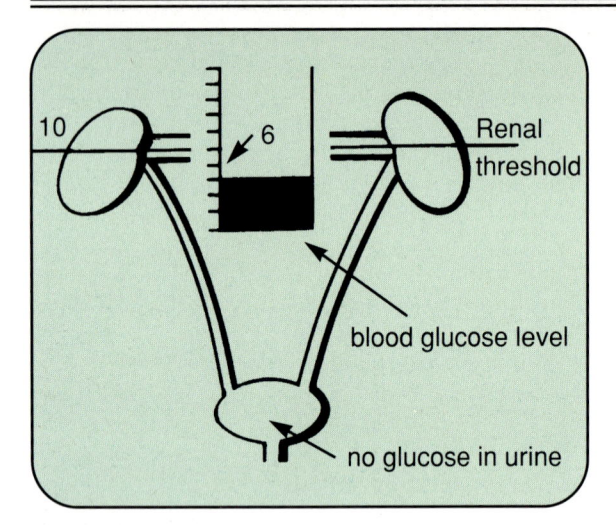

FIGURE 1: Usually the renal threshold is around 10 mmol/L. No glucose overflows into the urine.

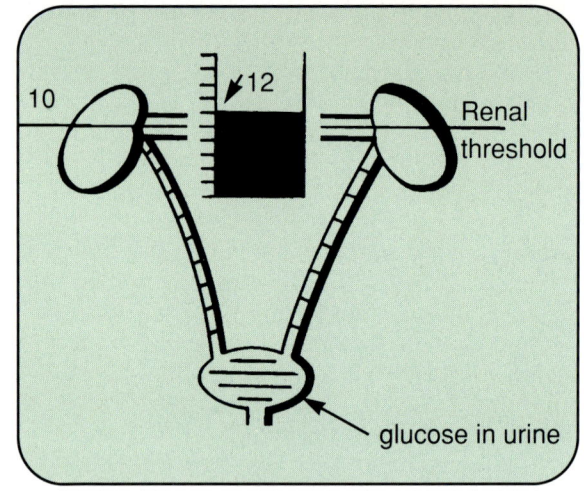

FIGURE 2: In diabetes the blood glucose may rise above the threshold. Glucose overflows into the urine.

There are a number of tablets and test strips available to measure for ketones, either specifically or along with glucose. Tests can be made for ketones with Ketostix, Keto-diastix (Ames) or Ketodiabur tablets (Boerhinger Mannheim) – all available from Diabetes Australia or pharmacies.

The doctor or diabetes nurse will explain how to use the testing system and advise which is best for any individual. The health professional will also explain the different characteristics of each product – for example, when using Ketodiastix, the presence of moderate to large amounts of ketones will give falsely low readings for glucose.

Testing for protein

Except during pregnancy, people with diabetes will rarely test their urine for protein, as the doctor usually does this for them.

The presence of more than a trace of protein suggests that the kidneys have been damaged in some way, such as the effects of many years of poor diabetic control and is therefore a bad sign.

This urine test is particularly important during pregnancy as the presence of protein may indicate the very serious condition of toxaemia of pregnancy.

This is not to say that the presence of protein always means kidney damage. It can merely indicate something such as an infection.

It has recently become possible to detect very small amounts of protein in the urine. These small amounts are referred to as "microalbuminuria". It has been shown that the continued presence of microalbuminuria indicates damage to the kidneys.

Both high blood pressure and poor control of diabetes produce microalbuminuria, but effective treatment of high blood pressure will reduce the amount of microalbuminuria, as does improved diabetic control.

People who are found to have microalbuminuria should therefore endeavour to achieve the best possible diabetic control and normal blood pressure.

The test for microalbuminuria is commonly performed in laboratories but tests are becoming available so that it can be performed in clinics, consulting rooms etc.

When to test

The person with diabetes must realise that the bladder is merely a storage depot and the urine in it could be a mixture of what has been stored there for two or more hours as well as

Testing Urine

some formed more recently. In this case the old urine could have glucose in it, and the newer urine no glucose, but the test would show glucose even though the blood level had already dropped back to normal. Because of this, there is no point testing urine from a full bladder.

The bladder should be emptied one and a half to two hours after a meal and test a specimen of urine about 15 to 30 minutes later. Sometimes it is more convenient to test just before the next meal.

Glucose from food increases blood glucose to its highest level after approximately one hour. The blood glucose level then falls progressively until the next meal. In other words, the lowest blood glucose level occurs before meals and the highest level one hour after meals. The value at two hours lies between these two.

Frequency of testing will vary from once daily to five or six times daily, depending on the circumstances.

For example, a person whose Type 2 diabetes is controlled by diet alone or diet plus tablets needs to test only once daily about two hours after a meal, choosing a different meal each day – after breakfast on day one, lunch on day two and so on.

These tests should prove negative for glucose but if not, more frequent urine testing must be carried out and the person should consult his or her doctor or diabetes nurse.

In the presence of some illness such as flu or bronchitis, the person with Type 2 diabetes will need to test urine as often as five or six times a day.

The preferable option for people with Type I or insulin dependent diabetes is to measure blood glucose, as urine testing is inaccurate. However if this is not possible they should test their urine at set times two or three times a day.

The information provided by two or three urine tests a day is often not enough when it comes to working out changes in insulin dosage. In order to establish a change in insulin dosage it may be necessary to have four or five urine tests a day – say, before breakfast, about two hours after breakfast, two hours after lunch, before the evening meal and about two hours after it.

These extra tests will probably be required for at least two weeks before any change in dosage is established.

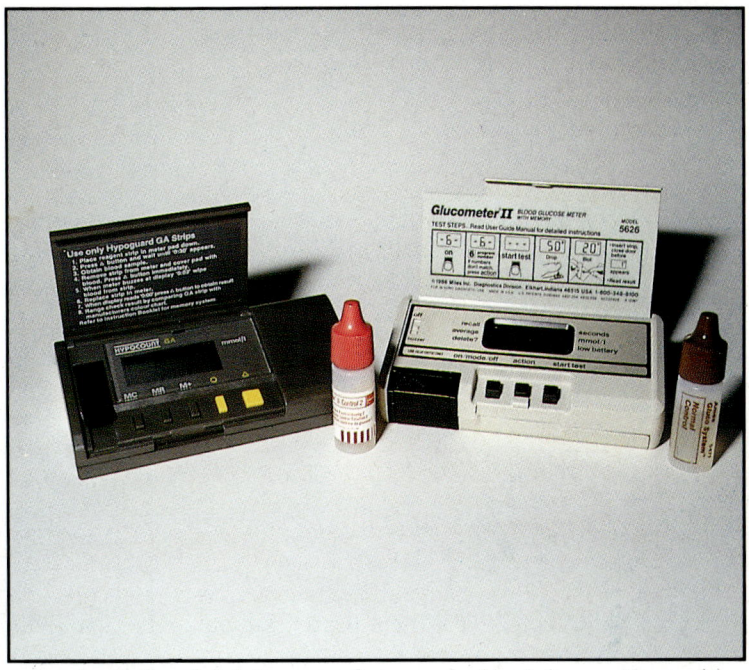

People with Type 1 diabetes may prefer to measure blood glucose with one of the modern blood glucose meters.

Interpreting the tests

The test before breakfast shows whether the previous day's insulin or tablet is working. The test before the evening meal measures the effect of that morning's medication and the other tests help fill in the picture throughout the previous 24 hours.

Recording results

Charts for recording results of urine tests are available in book form. Accurate records are needed to enable your doctor to make decisions on your treatment. The doctor will tell you the preferred method of recording the chart, either in colours, percentages, or "negative, trace, +, ++,+++,++++." ❑ ❑ ❑

Testing Urine

To the person who has just been diagnosed, or the parent of a child recently diagnosed as having diabetes, urine tests may sound complicated but this is not the case. In time they will become routine.

As with so many practices involved with diabetes, they should not be seen as an onerous task, but as a handy tool to help you take more control over your diabetes, and in turn, your life. Remember, these tests are your early warning system. Take notice of the signals they send.

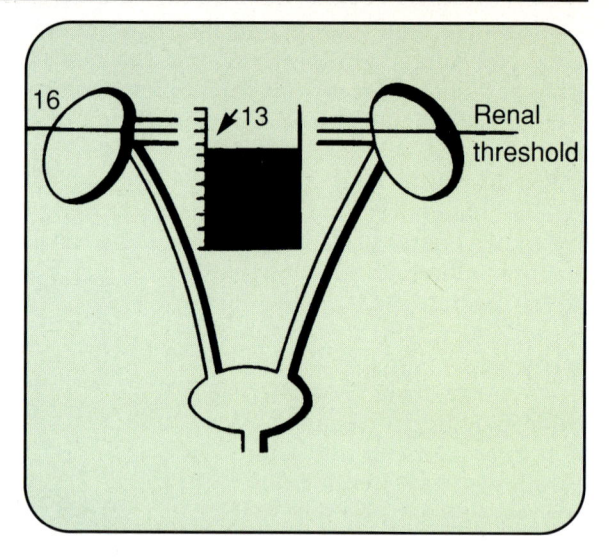

*FIGURE 3: **High renal threshold** – With a high renal threshold blood glucose levels can be higher than normal but no glucose overflows into the urine.*

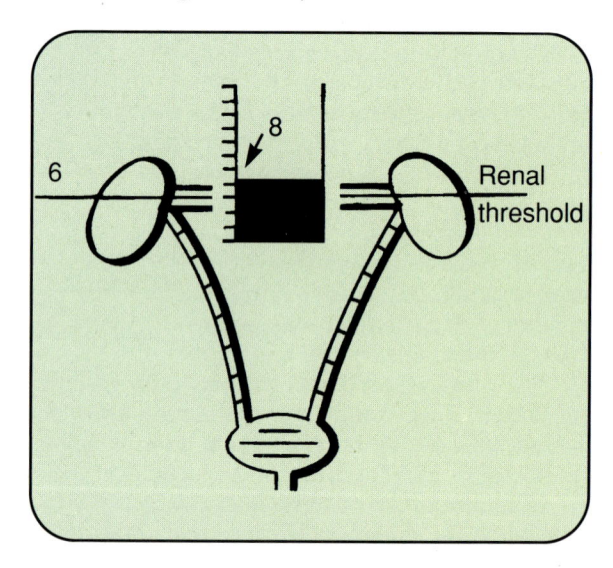

*FIGURE 4: **Low renal threshold** – With a low renal threshold blood glucose levels can be normal but glucose overflows into the urine.*

CHAPTER 11

Hypoglycaemia and Hyperglycaemia

By Dr Tim Welborn
Physician-in-Charge
Diabetes Clinic
Sir Charles Gairdner Hospital
Nedlands, W.A.

Hypoglycaemia means a low blood glucose level ("hypo" rhymes with "low"). People with Type 1 diabetes have to be particularly careful about low glucose levels, but some people with Type 2 diabetes on tablets can experience these effects also.

All people with diabetes will recognise the symptoms of high blood glucose levels, since these were present at the time of diagnosis.

This chapter describes the symptoms of low blood glucose and the symptoms of high blood glucose and how to treat these two separate problems.

Hypoglycaemia (Low Blood Glucose)

The symptoms of a low blood glucose level usually appear quite rapidly, over 10-15 minutes. It is important to recognise them because the remedy is very simple; that is, eating sugar or carbohydrate.

When the blood glucose level falls to less than 3.0mmol/L there are usually early warning symptoms. The brain sends messages to the adrenal glands which pour out adrenaline, causing:-
  A feeling of anxiety and unease.
  Palpitations or rapid heart beat.
  Sweating.
  Shakiness.
  Hunger.
  Pins and needles feeling round the mouth or in the hands.
These symptoms, which are adrenaline related, can occur with anxiety or apprehension (e.g. when going into a big examination, or about to face an important football match). These are the early warning symptoms of a falling blood glucose level and can usually be corrected promptly by taking sugar or some other form of carbohydrate by mouth.

If these symptoms are ignored or misinterpreted, or if there is unawareness of the early warning symptoms of low blood glucose it can progress to involve brain and nerve function. This is a more serious stage of hypoglycaemia and causes clumsiness, disturbed mood, such as irritability or aggressive behaviour or inappropriate responses. It is important for a relative or spouse to identify this stage because it can progress to coma or even epileptic convulsions unless treated promptly. In children the symptoms of hypoglycaemia may be overlooked since the child can show just irritability, aggressiveness, poor performance at school, excessive hunger, or unusual behaviour.

The most common causes of low blood glucose in a person with diabetes are as follows:-
- Lack of sufficient food intake.
- Too much insulin given.
- Excessive activity.
- Aiming at perfect diabetic control.
- Alcohol.

Insufficient food intake can be due to eating less or missing a meal, even not digesting the food properly (as can occur with the anxiety of a big examination). Sometimes excessive alcohol blunts awareness of the sympathetic warning to low blood glucose. Some patients are particularly susceptible to alcohol induced hypoglycaemia which stops their liver compensating.

Hypoglycaemia and Hyperglycaemia

	Hypoglycaemia (low blood glucose)	Hyperglycaemia (high blood glucose)
Cause	Too much insulin Too little food Food not digested (anxiety, nausea) Excessive exercise Alcohol.	Not enough insulin, or omission of insulin dose. Too much food Failure to test urine, or ignoring positive tests. Infections and illnesses. Injury and stress.
Onset	Good health immediately before. Rapid onset.	Ill health for hours or days. Gradual onset.
Symptoms and signs	Hunger, sweating, pallor, nervousness, headache, dizziness, palpitations. Tingling sensation in tongue and lips. Weakness. Progressing to:- Confusion, mood change, belligerence. Clumsiness, slurred speech. Drowsiness. Unconsciousness or coma. Convulsions and fitting.	Excessive thirst, excessive passage of large volumes of urine, dramatic weight-loss, weakness, lack of energy over a period of days. Progressing to:- Nausea and vomiting, abdominal pains, increased breathing. Smell of ketones (acetone) on breath. Drowsiness and dehydration. Unconsciousness or coma
Urine	Negative for glucose, providing the bladder has been recently emptied.	Glucose ++++ Large ketones
Blood	Low blood glucose, usually less than 3mmol/L.	High blood glucose higher than 15mmol/L.
Treatment	Immediate glucose, sweets, or sweet drinks by mouth. Alternatively carbohydrate food of any sort, biscuits, bananas etc. If uncooperative, try honey or syrup placed inside the cheek. Do not attempt to give solid foods by mouth. If unconscious, Glucagon injection either subcutaneously or into muscle will generally improve symptoms of hypoglycaemia in 10-15 min. If unconscious, lie on one side and ensure a good airway and lift the chin to enable more easy breathing. If fitting or convulsing, lie on one side, restrain excessive movements, prevent falls (from bed) until the fit subsides.	Test blood glucose levels every 2-4 hours and record the results. Test the urine for glucose and ketones. More than the normal dose of insulin is usually required. Seek advice concerning small doses of short-acting insulin, e.g. Soluble/Actrapid/Humulin R insulin 4 units every hour for adults subcutaneously. If vomiting occurs contact the doctor concerning treatment. Maintain at least the normal dose of insulin. If symptoms do not respond, hospitalisation is necessary as an emergency.

Glucagon is the first line of defence for a child.

Excessive insulin can occur through inadvertent overdosage (some people can give a double-dose without realising it), or just a natural mistake. Elderly people on tablets can have the same problem of missing meals or giving a double-dose of the medication.

Increased physical activity burns up blood glucose while the activity is in progress, but there is also an increased insulin sensitivity for 6-12 hours after very vigorous physical exertion.

Some people trying to get better control, e.g., the newly married woman who is wishing to have a baby, can be more prone to hypoglycaemia because her blood glucose levels are much lower and less warning occurs when blood glucose levels fall, e.g., from 5mmol/L to 3mmol/L.

The treatment of low blood glucose levels is very important and should be carefully studied by the person with diabetes and the people they live with and work with.

First of all, prevention is better than cure. All people on insulin should carry a supply of sugar, in the forms of glucose tablets, sugar lumps, jellybeans, or barley sugar, etc. These substances should be available in the car (if they drive) and in their drawer at work.

Early recognition of symptoms of hypoglycaemia by being alert to the symptoms described above will prevent progression to the more severe stages. Monitoring blood glucose levels is extremely helpful in this situation. It is especially important for people with diabetes who drive motor vehicles to be careful about identifying symptoms, and to check their blood glucose levels if in any doubt.

If hypoglycaemic symptoms are recognised or even just suspected, it is best to take action and treat!

Early symptoms can be treated by taking sugar by mouth, such as one or two dessertspoonfuls of glucose or table sugar, a can of ordinary lemonade or other sweet drink, biscuits, bread, a banana or honey.

Hypoglycaemia and Hyperglycaemia

This should cause improvement in 5-10 minutes. It is important then to take some long-acting carbohydrate such as bread or biscuit to be sure the improvement continues.

If symptoms have progressed to irritability or confusion – it is all the more important to get sugar into the person. Any reasonable method to encourage them to take something by mouth should be used. It can take half to one hour to recover fully, even if blood glucose levels come back to normal, and great care should be taken driving or working near machinery.

Finally, if the person is drowsy or goes into coma or has convulsions, this is clearly a medical emergency. An injection of glucagon (1 International Unit) can be given by a relative trained in the technique. The glucagon is given intramuscularly, into the muscles of the outer part of the thigh, but it works almost as quickly given subcutaneously (like insulin). Otherwise the best thing to do is to restrain the person from self-injury, lie them on one side, call an ambulance if possible, and get them to a Casualty or Emergency Centre. In hospital, emergency treatment can be given using an intravenous glucose injection.

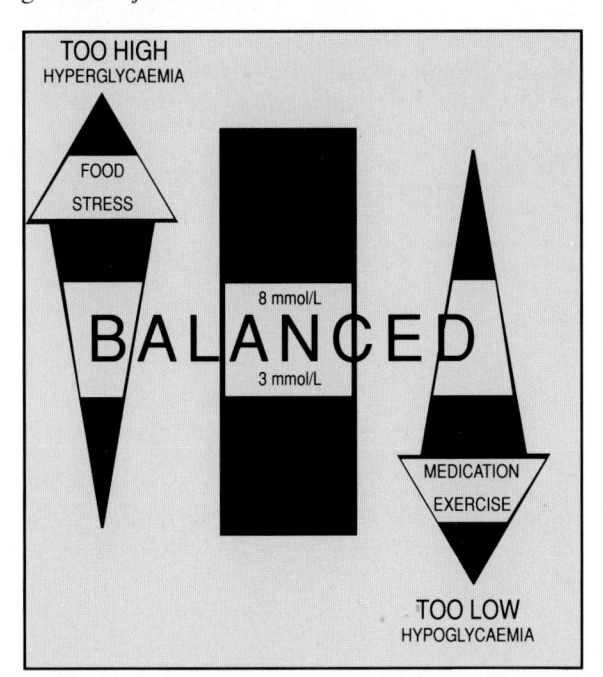

Repeated prolonged attacks of severe hypoglycaemia can cause nervous system injury and brain damage and should be avoided at all costs.

Most people on insulin, and some on tablets, will have experienced mild hypoglycaemia at times. With the introduction of human insulin, an increasing number of people claim that there is no good early warning and they go straight into confusion or slurred speech or other disturbed brain function symptoms. Thus it is all the more important for these people to monitor their blood glucose levels regularly, and to be particularly attentive to mealtimes and snacktimes.

GLUCAGON

Glucagon is a protein made by the pancreas. Just as insulin pulls the blood glucose down, glucagon pushes the blood glucose up. This "push pull" control keeps blood glucose stable in people without diabetes.

In people with diabetes, glucagon is useful to push the blood glucose up when too much exercise, insulin or medication have pulled it down too far and the person can't or won't take sugar or food.

In this case, glucagon can be injected and will push glucose out from stores in the liver and in to the blood. Then the person will become cooperative and can eat something.

Glucagon comes as a dry powder to be mixed with a fluid. The idea is to mix the fluid with the powder (swirl, don't shake), inject the glucagon as you would insulin and rub vigorously.

The glucagon usually takes several minutes to work. In the meantime, make sure the person is lying safely on their side and that the airways are clear. If you are not sure how to do this, go to a First-Aid Course. When the person awakes, food should be given and you should make sure someone goes with the person, in case the hypo comes back.

The last point is to remember to ask WHY the hypo happened and to take necessary precautions (including getting new glucagon stocks).

TOO HIGH — HYPERGLYCAEMIA
FOOD / STRESS

BALANCED
8 mmol/L
3 mmol/L

MEDICATION / EXERCISE
TOO LOW — HYPOGLYCAEMIA

HYPERGLYCAEMIA

The onset of hyperglycaemia is much more gradual and can take hours or days. Most people with diabetes will know of the symptoms of very high blood glucose level:

Extreme thirst.
Passage of large volumes of urine frequently.
Weight loss.
Weakness.
Blurred vision.

If the person has Type 1 diabetes, with no insulin secretion of his/her own, severe hyperglycaemia can become even more serious with the following manifestations:

Ketones on the breath.
Deep breathing.
Abdominal pain.
Drowsiness.
Coma.

On the other hand, many people with diabetes can have mild hyperglycaemia recognisable by some dryness of the mouth, passing urine once or twice overnight, indolent skin infections or genital irritation, and unusual tiredness.

Causes of hyperglycaemia are insufficient insulin, either a mistaken dosage, or not giving the injection, or that the insulin has "gone off" for some reason or other (in Type 1 diabetes), and forgetting to take the usual tablets (in Type 2 diabetes). Dietary indiscretions are a common cause. Infection or other intercurrent illness can precipitate hyperglycaemia. Mental stress may activate brain mechanisms that work against insulin's action and cause high blood glucose levels most of the time. Some people have true insulin resistance requiring very large doses of insulin and this often requires careful testing in the hospital situation.

Severe hyperglycaemia in people with Type 1 diabetes must be recognised and the insulin dosage increased. If necessary ring your doctor or nurse about this. It is usually quite safe to give frequent small doses of short acting insulin, 4-8 units every hour as required, by subcutaneous injection. If you know how to give intramuscular injections, small doses of short acting insulin every hour are very effective (important – see Chapter 13, Sick Days). Hyperglycaemia in someone with Type 2 diabetes on tablets is often temporary and although the dose of tablets is sometimes increased this is not always effective. Medical advice should be sought if symptoms persist.

Intake of fluids is very important where there are symptoms of high blood glucose. Drink as much water or low calorie fluids as possible to keep up with the fluid that is lost by passing urine. Don't take fluids that contain sugar because this will make the symptoms and the

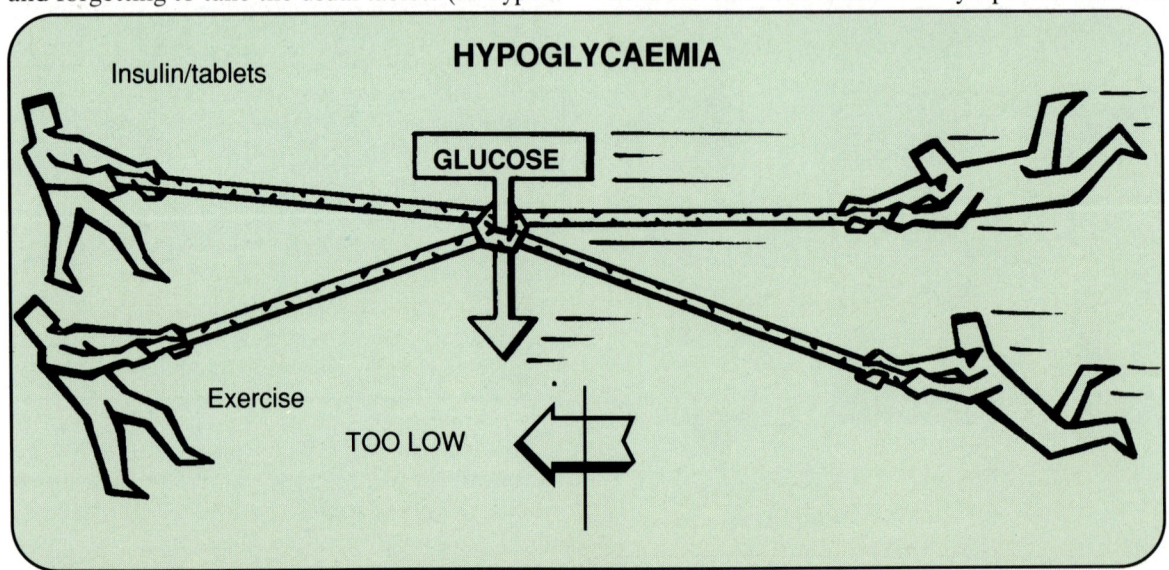

HYPOGLYCAEMIA

Insulin/tablets
GLUCOSE
Exercise
TOO LOW

HYPERGLYCAEMIA

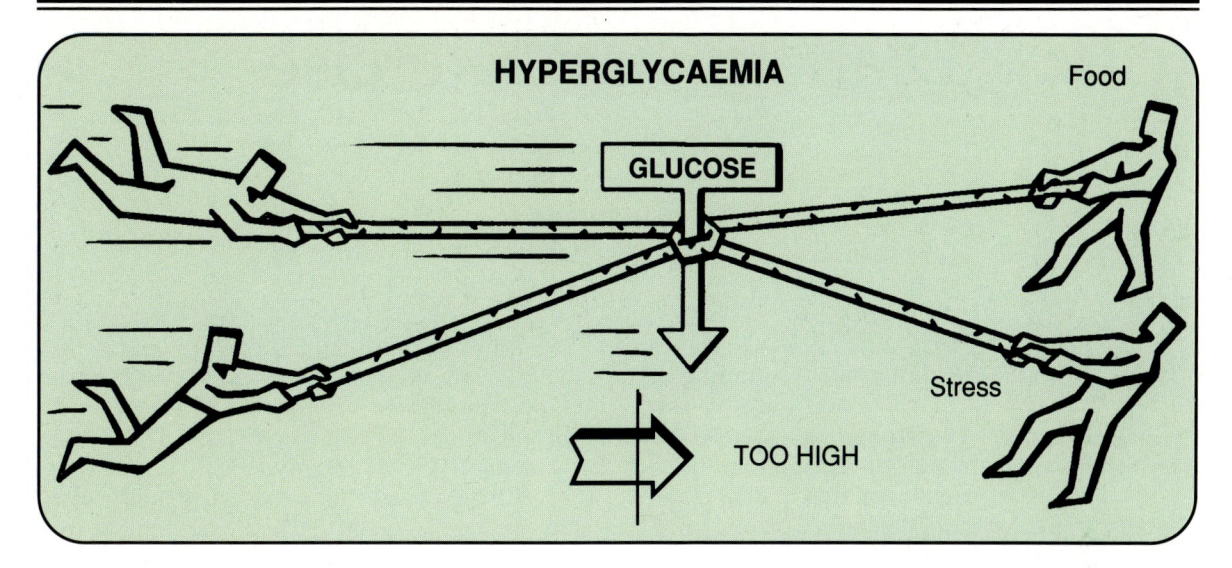

Food

Stress

GLUCOSE → TOO HIGH

hyperglycaemia much worse.

If vomiting prevents fluid intake and makes eating difficult, this is a real emergency, and a doctor should be notified. An injection can be given to stop the vomiting reflex.

❑ ❑ ❑

This chapter has dealt mainly with the emergency treatment of hypoglycaemia and hyperglycaemia. Lesser degrees of low and high blood glucose levels can exist in people with diabetes and cause unrecognised problems. It is important therefore to check blood glucose profiles at regular intervals and to have these on record when you visit your doctor or diabetes nurse. This gives the best chance of you being able to discuss management and obtaining useful advice. Measurement of somewhat low blood glucose levels before breakfast or before lunch can give "early warning" that the insulin dosage should be adjusted. Similarly, many people run rather high blood glucose levels putting them at risk of complications (see the separate chapter on this). In such people, adjustment of insulin and fine tuning ("the right insulin at the right time") should help them get back on the tramlines.

CHAPTER 12

Diabetes and Exercise

By Prof. Don Chisholm
Head, Metabolic Division,
Garvan Institute
of Medical Research

An understanding of the relationship between diabetes and exercise is of great importance in the proper management of diabetes for two main reasons.

Firstly, it is important that people with diabetes who wish to play sport or engage in vigorous physical activity are able to do so without running into serious problems and secondly, there is evidence to suggest that regular physical activity may have important benefits for the person with diabetes.

As far as those benefits are concerned, one of the major metabolic defects associated with diabetes is a poor response of the body's tissues to insulin, called insulin resistance.

It has now been clearly demonstrated that regular physical activity can improve insulin sensitivity or to some extent reverse insulin resistance.

Studies suggest people who have a relatively active lifestyle have only about half the chance of developing Type 2 (non-insulin dependent) diabetes as those who are physically inactive. Moreover, regular physical activity assists in weight reduction which is of paramount importance in the management of Type 2 diabetes.

Therefore it is appropriate to regard exercise as a very important component of therapy in Type 2 diabetes.

Insulin resistance is not a major feature of Type 1 (insulin dependent) diabetes. It is therefore generally not expected that regular exercise will reverse the metabolic abnormality of Type 1 diabetes. However, regular physical activity may lead to a reduced insulin dosage as well as cardiovascular benefits.

In both types of diabetes there is a substantially increased risk of coronary artery disease and disease of other blood vessels in the body.

Regular physical activity has a number of effects which might be expected to reduce the risk of cardiovascular disease – such as a reduction in the bad type of cholesterol (LDL cholesterol) or an increase in the good type of cholesterol (HDL cholesterol), reduced blood pressure and a reduction in the clotting elements of the blood (aggregation of platelets).

Although there is no absolute proof that regular physical activity over many years reduces cardiovascular risk in people with diabetes, there is a lot of indirect evidence to suggest that this is the case. Therefore most diabetes physicians would feel that regular exercise is a desirable objective in the management of diabetes.

What happens during exercise in people without diabetes?

Exercise is a very profound stimulus to glucose utilisation. During moderate exercise, the amount of glucose being used up by the body increases by 200 – 300 per cent.

Obviously with so much glucose being used, if there were no compensating mechanism, the blood glucose level would fall dramatically during exercise. However, the liver, in response to messages transmitted by hormones and from the nervous system, increases its production of glucose to exactly correspond to the amount of glucose being used.

Therefore people without diabetes can exercise for up to about two hours without taking any glucose or carbohydrate and without any significant fall in their blood glucose level.

Diabetes and Exercise

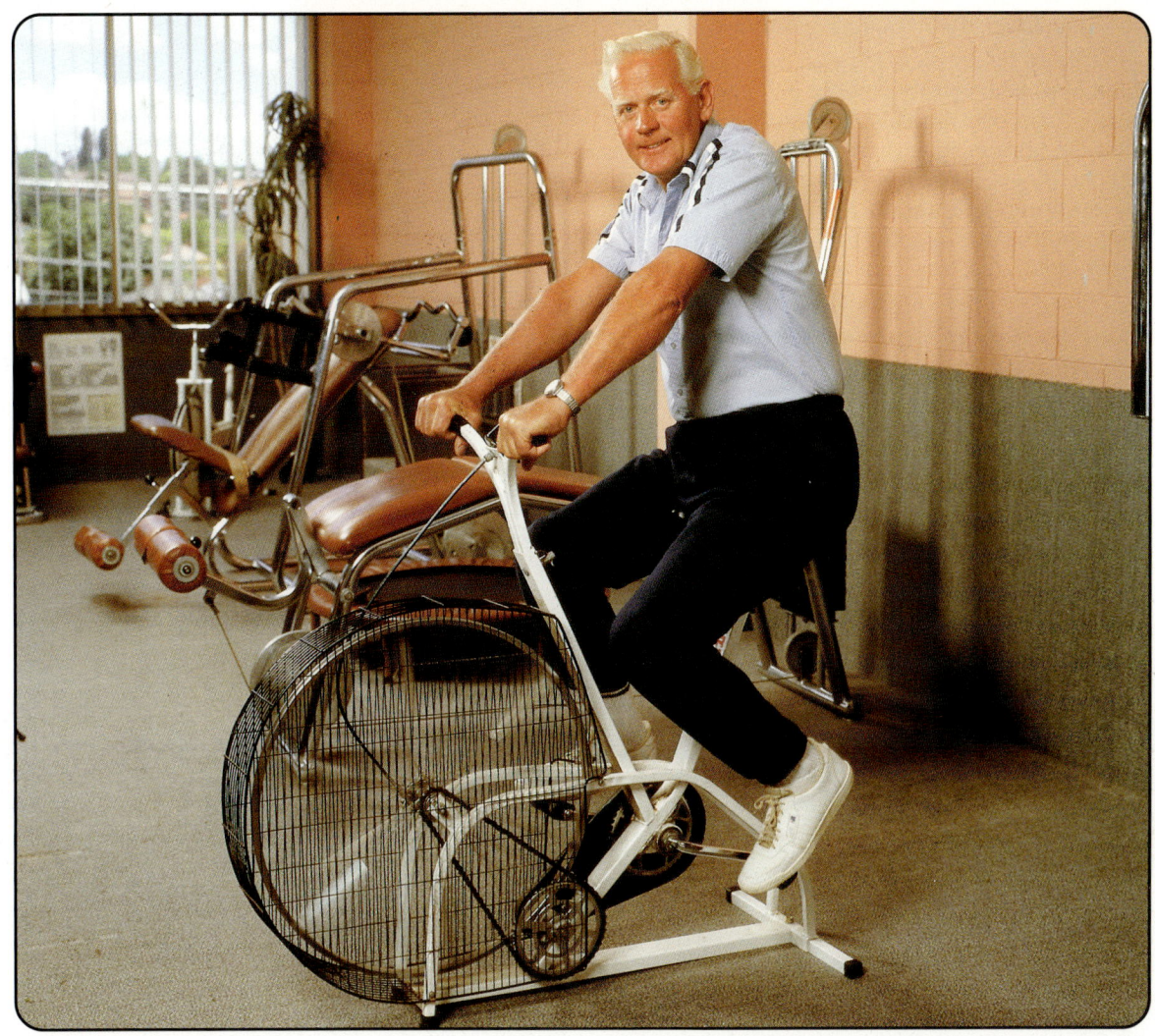

The other important thing about exercise is that it greatly increases the response of the exercising muscles, and of the whole body, to insulin. In other words, it increases the body's insulin sensitivity. This effect is produced for about 12 hours by a single bout of exercise and for a much longer time with regular exercise training.

It is this effect which is believed to be of benefit in both the prevention and treatment of Type 2 diabetes.

What happens in people with diabetes?

The effect of exercise on people with diabetes is the same as in people without diabetes – the glucose usage by muscles increases.

The difference is that the response of the liver is much more unpredictable in people with diabetes. Commonly the liver puts out less glucose than is used by muscles. Therefore the blood glucose level falls.

This is not always the case though and the liver may put out the same amount of glucose as is used by the muscles or even more. Of course if the liver puts out more glucose than is used by muscles the blood glucose level will rise – as sometimes happens during exercise in people with diabetes.

Diabetes and Exercise

How to manage diabetes during exercise

It must be emphasised that the response of blood glucose levels to exercise in diabetes varies greatly from one individual to another. Thus the following advice is appropriate when initiating an exercise program but it is very important for each person with diabetes to determine their own response to exercise, and to modify their intake of carbohydrates, insulin or tablets accordingly.

Some common management principles are:

Intake of extra carbohydrates before and during exercise

For people with diabetes who are taking insulin injections or sulphonylurea tablets there is a high probability of a substantial fall in the blood glucose level during exercise. Therefore extra complex carbohydrates should be taken 30-60 minutes before exercise or extra simple sugars immediately before or during exercise.

The usual advice is to take about 15 grams of carbohydrate (equivalent to one slice of bread or one third of a can of ordinary lemonade) for each 20 minutes of exercise of moderate severity – such as brisk walking which makes the person breathe heavily but would allow them to carry on a conversation with a few puffs between sentences.

For exercise lasting more than an hour it is unwise to try to take all the carbohydrate beforehand so the person should have some ordinary lemonade or other simple sugar to take at regular intervals during the exercises.

Although the blood glucose response to exercise varies greatly from one individual to another, it tends to follow the same pattern for a person doing the same exercise at the same time of day.

This means the blood glucose level should be checked after exercise to enable a management plan to be worked out. If it has risen substantially by the end of the exercise, it would be appropriate to take a little less carbohydrate on the next occasion. Conversely, if the blood glucose was unduly low at the end of exercise it would be appropriate to take a little more carbohydrate on the next occasion.

In people who are not on insulin but are taking sulphonylurea tablets there is a risk that exercise will cause a substantial reduction of glucose with the possibility of a hypoglycaemic reaction. However the fall in blood glucose is likely to be substantially less than in people taking insulin.

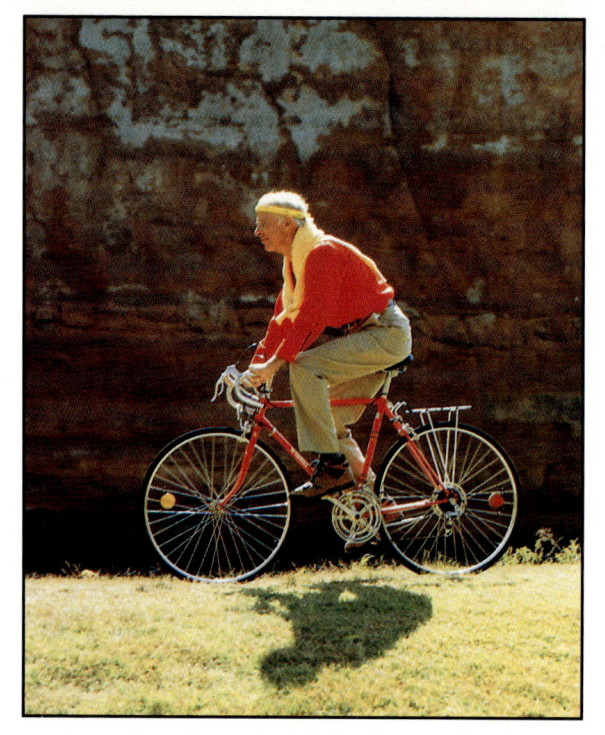

People with Type 2 diabetes on tablets are also often trying to lose weight, therefore it would be reasonable to take only half the amount of extra carbohydrate suggested earlier during exercise and monitor the blood glucose response. If there is a substantial fall in blood glucose it may be better to reduce the sulphonylurea tablet dosage when exercising than increase carbohydrate intake.

Adjustment of Insulin Dosage

If exercise is of relatively brief duration, it is often best not to make any adjustment of the insulin dosage and to deal with the situation entirely by dietary adjustment. If exercise is more prolonged it is usually desirable to reduce the dose of insulin operating at the time of exercise as well as taking extra food.

Once again one must keep in mind that the

response to exercise is very variable from one individual to another. It is therefore important to determine the blood glucose response in each individual and to modify the reduction in insulin according to the response.

Adjustment of tablet therapy

In people taking only metformin tablets there is virtually no risk of a hypoglycaemic or low blood glucose reaction, therefore it is usually appropriate to continue the same tablet dosage.

For people taking sulphonylurea tablets (e.g. Daonil, Diamicron, Minidiab, Rastinon, Diabinese etc) there is a potential risk of a substantial fall in blood glucose during exercise. This may be prevented by extra carbohydrate intake with exercise as indicated earlier. However if the patient is trying to lose weight and wants to avoid extra food intake, it may be reasonable to reduce the dose of sulphonylurea tablet on the morning of the day of exercise.

Once again it is important to check the blood glucose response and to modify the diet or tablet adjustment until a satisfactory blood glucose response is achieved.

Late Hypoglycaemia Occurring After Exercise

As mentioned previously, a single bout of exercise may improve the body's insulin sensitivity for about 12 hours afterwards.

This means there is real risk of a hypoglycaemic reaction occurring in the 12 hours after exercise in patients taking insulin treatment. This risk is quite substantial in people with Type 1 diabetes but is not so pronounced in people who have Type 2 diabetes who are on insulin treatment or sulphonylurea tablets.

It is quite common for someone with Type 1 diabetes who plays a long game of tennis in the afternoon to get a hypoglycaemic reaction around midnight to 2am. Therefore it is usually wise to make a small reduction in the dosage of insulin operating during the 12 hours after vigorous exercise.

In other words, the person playing a long game of tennis in the afternoon would probably be wise to make a 10-20 per cent reduction in the evening doses of quick and intermediate acting insulin to avoid night-time hypoglycaemia.

Once again there is a lot of variation from one individual to another and insulin adjustment should be modified once the blood glucose response has been determined on the first couple of occasions.

Additional Advice With Regard to Insulin or Sulphonylurea Tablets

If an insulin injection is given into a limb which is going to be vigorously exercised, the insulin will be absorbed into the bloodstream more rapidly during the exercise. This increases the risk of hypoglycaemia, therefore it is wise not to inject insulin into an arm or leg that is going to be involved in the exercise. In general, injecting into the abdominal wall is best when exercise is planned.

Be careful about exercise when the blood glucose level is already high. If the insulin dosage prior to exercise is reduced too much, or if some other problem has caused a rise in blood glucose so that the blood glucose level is already substantially elevated when exercise is commenced there may be a very adverse response to exercise.

In particular when a person starts exercise with his/her diabetes under poor control there may be a greater rise in blood glucose levels and a substantial increase in ketones.

If very prolonged vigorous exercise is planned such as marathon running or triathlons, it may be necessary to make a much more substantial reduction in the morning dose of insulin. Sometimes it is necessary to reduce the insulin dose to less than half of the usual amount. People who undertake this sort of activity usually do a lot of training for the event – so the degree of insulin reduction can be worked out over a period of time as their response to the exercise is determined.

Other important considerations

Recognition of Hypoglycaemia

During exercise it may be more difficult to recognise the warning symptoms of hypoglycaemia. Warning symptoms like sweating,

Diabetes and Exercise

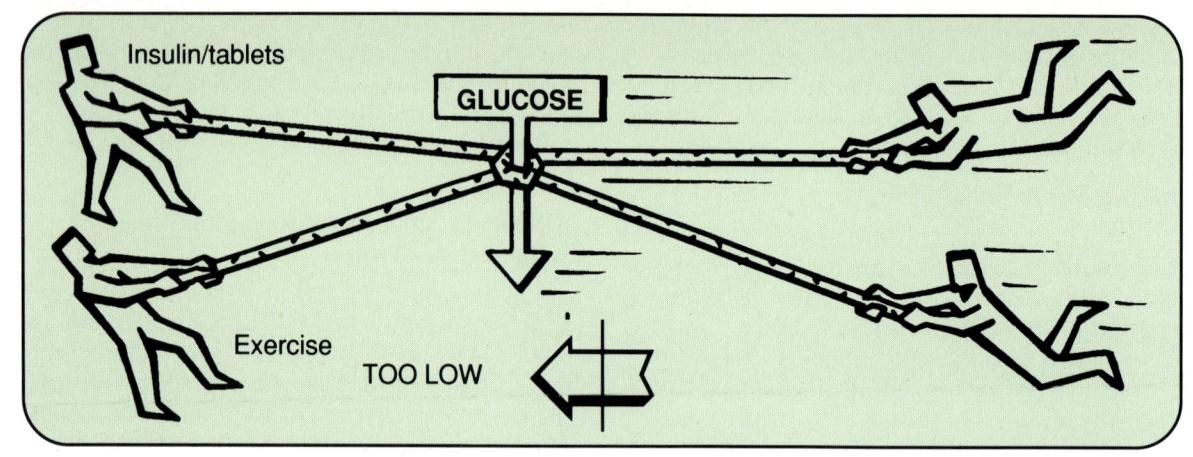

palpitations, tremulousness may be confused with the responses to exercise itself.

Because of this, it is very important that people with diabetes who are exercising (especially those with Type 1 diabetes) are very careful to take the necessary steps to avoid hypoglycaemia- and that they take special care to immediately take some sugar if they do notice any of the warning symptoms of a hypoglycaemic reaction. Don't forget to always carry sugar in your pocket.

Need to Reduce Dosage of Insulin or Sulphonylurea Tablets

When people increase their amount of regular physical activity, their response to insulin or sulphonylurea tablets tends to increase. This means it is often necessary to reduce the dosage of insulin or sulphonylurea tablets to avoid hypoglycaemia.

Risk of Coronary Artery Disease

People with diabetes have an increased risk of coronary artery disease. Therefore it is very important that people with diabetes who are over the age of about 35 have a cardiovascular assessment prior to any substantial increase in their level of physical activity.

Depending on the circumstances of the individual this assessment may be a simple clinical examination, or could include an electrocardiograph or a cardiac stress test.

Foot Problems

Ulcers or other lesions on the feet are a great potential danger in people with diabetes and so it is vitally important that people with diabetes who are planning to increase their regular physical activity do so in a way that does not cause damage to their feet. This is particularly true for middle aged and elderly people and in fact it is often wise for them to avoid exercises such as running, which causes a lot of stress to the feet.

Exercise which poses minimal weight or stress on the feet, such as riding an exercise bike, is ideal – although brisk walking in good footwear could also be an excellent form of exercise.

It is usually wise for someone in the middle age group or older to have an assessment from a podiatrist regarding the state of their feet and the most desirable type of footwear before embarking on an exercise program.

Exercise in People with Retinopathy

In any person who has diabetes with actively progressing retinopathy, exercise may present some danger as it could cause bleeding from blood vessels in the back of the eye. Sudden stress anaerobic exercises like weight lifting are more dangerous than aerobic exercises like jogging. However it is wise to avoid any vigorous exercise until the eye specialist indicates that laser therapy or other treatment has arrested the progression of the retinopothy, and it is in a stable state.

Diabetes and Exercise

What type of exercise?

Aerobic Versus Non-Aerobic Physical Activity

Aerobic activity is the term relating to exercise which is associated with movement over a reasonably long period during which the body uses a substantial amount of oxygen, such as jogging or swimming. Aerobic activity is generally beneficial to the body and causes improvements in insulin sensitivity, blood pressure and lipids.

Anaerobic physical activity is usually a sudden, rapid stressful exercise such as weight lifting or 100 metre sprints. This type of activity is believed to cause less benefit and may be associated with a sharp rise in blood pressure. It is generally thought not to be a desirable type of exercise for people with diabetes.

Activities Which May Present Special Dangers

Because of the risk of a hypoglycaemic reaction causing mental confusion or coma, there are certain activities which may constitute a major danger to people with insulin treated diabetes – such as motor racing, high standard mountain climbing, hang gliding, solo yachting or scuba diving. It is generally felt that these activities should be avoided.

Other activities which also have some potential danger may be undertaken as long as the person recognises and accepts the risks. With these activities it is highly desirable that the person with diabetes undertakes the activity in the company of a "buddy" who understands about the person's diabetes and knows how to deal with a hypoglycaemic reaction. Such activities might include surfboard riding, long distance running, triathlons or cross-country skiing.

How much exercise is desirable?

There has not been enough study of the long term effects of exercise in people with diabetes to give a precise answer to this question but 20 to 40 minutes of moderate exercise, three or four times a week has been shown to be very useful in exerting favourable effects on lipids, blood pressure and cardiac function Therefore this is suggested as the ideal, however some recent studies suggest that lesser amounts of physical activity may still have important beneficial effects with regard to cardiovascular disease.

Moderate physical activity means exercise that is sufficiently strenuous to make the person puff a bit; but they would be able to carry on a conversation with someone during exercise, taking a few puffs between sentences. This is about 50 per cent of maximum aerobic capacity.

❑ ❑ ❑

In summary, with appropriate precautions it is possible for nearly all people with diabetes to engage in regular physical activity and to participate in most sporting activities however it is very important that the appropriate precautions are taken to avoid hypoglycaemic or hyperglycaemic problems.

In this regard self blood glucose monitoring is vital to make appropriate adjustment in diet and medications and to maintain blood glucose control during and after exercise.

It is extremely important that people in middle age or in an older age group have an assessment regarding cardiovascular risk and foot complications, before they undertake an exercise program. However if a gradual and sensible approach is taken even people who have some complications of diabetes may safely undertake regular physical activity.

TIPS FOR EXERCISE

- Take extra carbohydrate before and during
- Adjust insulin and medication
- Take care of feet.

CHAPTER 13

Sick Days

By Clin. Assoc. Professor Paul Moffitt
and Melba Mensch
Royal Newcastle Hospital
Newcastle

Monitoring blood and urine

Testing the blood and urine for glucose is never more important than on a day of sickness or injury. The tests should be performed at least every four hours and, if glucose is present in high concentrations, as frequently as hourly. It is absolutely essential for people with diabetes to test for the presence of ketones in the urine and the frequency of testing throughout the day will depend upon the presence or absence of ketones as well as upon the level of blood glucose.

A trace of ketones in the urine is commonly found in people who are dieting or who are feeling too ill to eat and is not a cause for alarm. However, in both Type 1 and Type 2 diabetes, a test should be undertaken again in two hours in order to determine that the concentration of ketones is not increasing. The presence of moderate or strong ketones in the urine is an ominous sign and medical assistance should immediately be sought and this becomes even more urgent if the patient is vomiting.

Insulin or Tablets

The human body's reaction to infection, sickness or injury is to increase its production of defensive hormones. These hormones increase the pulse rate, perspiration and release glucose into the blood stream from stores in the liver. The hormones also render insulin less effective in removing glucose from the blood.

The effect of illness on a person with diabetes is therefore a rise in blood glucose. You can imagine what would happen if the sick or injured person with diabetes did not take his/her usual dose of insulin or tablets – the blood glucose would go even higher and higher.

It is imperative for you to understand that the blood glucose level of a person with diabetes may indeed rise on a sick day even though no food or glucose containing drink has been taken. It is equally important to understand that although insulin taken without food will produce hypoglycaemia in the healthy person with diabetes, the same injection of insulin is unlikely to produce hypoglycaemia when that person is ill or injured.

There is no guarantee however that the insulin taken on a day of illness will not produce hypoglycaemia and this is one of the reasons why it is necessary for the blood to be tested at least every four hours.

But, there is a second problem. Another of insulin's actions is to restrain the body from converting its own fat into ketones. Small amounts of ketones are commonly seen during dieting and sometimes after hypoglycaemia and are of no consequence.

When ketones are present in high concentrations in the blood they are highly toxic and the state of diabetic keto-acidosis develops. Keto-acidosis can lead to death and it is important that it is prevented from occurring.

It is therefore essential for people with Type 1 diabetes to have their usual dose of insulin, not only to prevent the blood glucose from rising, but to prevent keto-acidosis occurring.

It is equally important for people with Type 2 diabetes who have been converted to insulin, to take the usual insulin dosage on a day of illness or injury.

People on tablets for Type 2 diabetes are similarly at risk of high blood glucose levels and must take their normal tablets. Because they do secrete some insulin of their own, people with Type 2 diabetes do not usually develop keto-acidosis.

Sick Days

Extra Insulin

Additional or increased doses of insulin given in the home can frequently avert hospitalisation. The additional insulin used is short-acting such as Actrapid or Humulin R given once daily or more often as single injections equal to 10-20 per cent of the normal total dosage per day. The dosage given, the frequency and route of injection will depend upon the circumstances prevailing in that particular person at that particular time. The factors to be taken into consideration are: the height of the blood glucose; the person's age; the total insulin dosage taken on a normal day; the presence or absence of ketones in the urine; the response to a previously given extra injection.

Sometimes it is necessary to give the extra insulin into the muscle rather than into the fat as the absorption of insulin from muscle is much more rapid than it is from the fat.

Let us look at some examples:

> *Suppose a 12 year-old boy normally receives Actrapid 6 units, Protaphane 18 units prior to breakfast with 8 units of each prior to the evening meal If, on a day when he has "the flu" he is found to have a blood glucose level in excess of 20 mmol/L with no ketones in the urine on two occasions three hours apart then he should receive more short-acting insulin (in addition to his normal insulin which had already been taken.)*
>
> *He could therefore be given 4 units of Actrapid (10 per cent of 40 units) subcutaneously. He would then be given no further insulin or four units or eight units four hours later, dependent upon whether there had been a marked fall in his blood glucose, a moderate fall or an increase.*

Suppose that the same boy has a blood glucose level of 24 mmol/L with a trace of ketones in his urine. In this case he would be given 10 per cent of his normal total insulin (four units) as Actrapid subcutaneously or into a muscle. He should then be tested again two hours later and the same dosage or a 50 per cent increase (six units) given if the blood glucose had not fallen. This could be repeated two hours later. However, the occurrence of vomiting or an increase in ketones in the urine in the meantime would be an indication for an urgent medical consultation or admission to hospital.

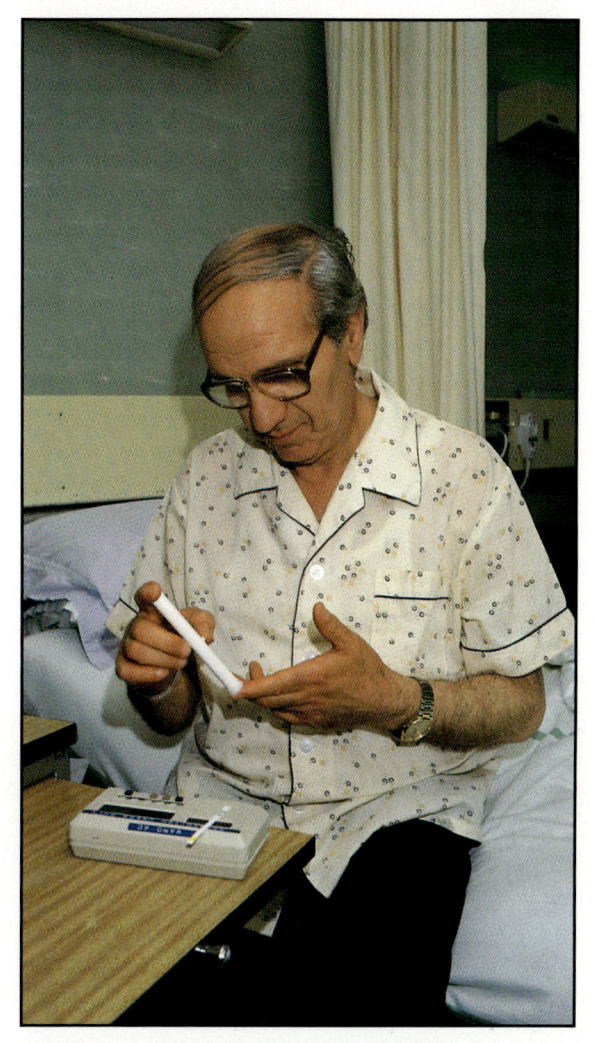

A person whose usual insulin is a short-acting insulin prior to each meal with a basal long-acting insulin given at some other time would increase the short-acting insulin dosage or dosages but leave the long-acting insulin unchanged.

An example could be a person receiving 6 units of Humulin R before each meal with 22 units of Humulin UL at 10pm. The total insulin dosage being 40 units this person could increase

Sick Days

Sick Day Diet Chart (6500 Kj)

(15 g carbohydrate exchanges/portions)

Breakfast (3 Exchanges/portions)

¾ cup orange juice
2 slices toast
(If unable to eat both slices of toast – wait 1-2 hours and have a ½ cup fruit juice instead)

Morning tea (1 Exchange/portion)

½ cup apple juice or
2 Saos if tolerated
Butter, Vegemite or cheese may be added if desired

Lunch (3 Exchanges/portions)

¾ cup soup (commercial or home-made)
1 slice bread
3/4 cup orange juice or soft canned or fresh fruit

Afternoon tea (l Exchange/portion)

Plain biscuit and ¼ cup pineapple juice

Tea (3 Exchanges/portions)

¾ cup soup
Low fat meat, fish, egg if tolerated
½ cup potato or 1 slice bread
½ cup ice cream or sweetened custard or fruit juice

Supper (l Exchange/portion)

½ English muffin or 1 slice toast
or
½ cup apple juice

The following foods could be added if desired:

Low fat meats, fish, chicken, cheese or egg
Margarine, peanut butter
Low joule spreads such as Vegemite, low joule jams

When vomiting, diarrhoea or fever occurs, it is necessary to replace salt and fluids Therefore, try to have some extra:

Bonox, Bovril, clear broth, salty soup, AND other fluids

---

the Humulin R dosages by four to eight units or have the extra units between the normal pre-meal injections. This would equally apply to any other person with a similar combination of short-acting and intermediate or long-acting insulins. (See Chapter 7, Types of Insulin).

> *Let us suppose that a 42-year-old woman normally receives Humulin-R 6 units Humulin-NPH 20 units before breakfast and Humulin-R 4 units Humulin-NPH 10 units before the evening meal. At midday on a day of illness she finds that her blood glucose, which was 14 mmol/L before breakfast, is 20 mmol/L even though she had her normal morning insulin. Her urine contains no ketones. She then takes 10 per cent of her total daily insulin (four units) as the short-acting insulin Humulin-R subcutaneously. At 4pm her blood sugar is still 20 mmol/L and again her urine does not contain ketones. Another Humulin-R 4 units is taken followed by her normal evening insulin just prior to the evening meal. If unable to eat she would take her normal evening intermediate acting insulin (Humulin-NPH) at its normal time and continue to test fourth hourly.*

If the same lady had been receiving a mixed insulin such as 26 units of Mixtard 30/70 prior to breakfast and 14 units prior to the evening meal, she would not be in a position to give herself extra short-acting insulin. She could however increase her evening Mixtard by up to 20 per cent of the total daily insulin dosage. She could therefore give herself as much as eight extra units bringing her total evening insulin dosage to Mixtard 22 units.

A person receiving a once daily injection of a single or pre-mixed insulin could increase the dosage on the second or later days by 20 per cent if higher than normal blood glucose levels persist, eg Humulin-NPH or Mixtard 40 units could become 48 units. Another person who mixes his/her own insulin could have one or more additional doses of the short acting insulin later in the day as described above, eg the usual Actrapid 6 Monotard 24 prior to breakfast with Actrapid 3 to 6 units later in the day.

Sick Days

A small number of people with Type 1 and 2 diabetes receiving insulin do not measure their own blood glucose but rely on urine tests to indicate the degree of glucose in their blood. This is a very inaccurate way of estimating the blood glucose and therefore extra insulin cannot be given merely because a urine test indicates maximum glucose in the urine. The presence of ketones as well however would necessitate further insulin as would the persistence of maximum glucose in the urine over six hours.

Even the most knowledgeable of patients would be wise not to give a third additional injection of insulin without seeking medical advice. Less knowledgeable patients should discuss the administration of any additional insulin with their medical practitioner.

The person with Type 2 diabetes who is normally controlled by diet alone or diet plus tablets may require insulin during an illness and particularly with surgery. The presence of maximum glucose in the urine over a period of six hours with or without ketones being present requires a medical consultation.

The first essential for an infant, child or adult is **take your usual insulin or tablet** (if you vomit the tablet ask for medical advice).

Food and drink

People with nausea or loss of appetite should endeavour to eat or drink the equivalent of his or her usual carbohydrate intake providing that the blood glucose level is not already more than 10 mmol/L. This could be achieved by frequent small meals or drinks. Foods suitable for the sick person include ice cream, eggs or egg flips, sweet biscuits soaked in milk or tea, bread, fruit and drinks such as lemonade, coca cola, ginger ale, fruit juices, broths and thick soups. Bananas contain potassium which is very important to the human body and is lost in the urine during illnesses. Broths also are of great value as they supply the salt which the sick person loses in perspiration and urine.

The chart, **Food for Sick Days** lists a large number of foods which are easily digestible by the sick person. Each is equal to the other and are equivalent to 1 carbohydrate exchange.

Minimum fluid intake for different age groups	
Age	Volume/kg per day
0-6 months	150 to 200 ml
6-12 months	120 to 150 ml
1-5 years	100ml
6-10 years	70ml
Over 10 years	50-60ml

Additional fluid will be needed to meet fluid losses during fever, vomiting and diarrhoea.

The **sick day diet chart** for the person who is normally receiving 6,500Kj (1500 cal.) diet. People receiving higher Kj diets need only to proportionally increase this diet to comply with their own.

Dehydration is a life threatening condition which can occur rapidly in any sick diabetic child or adult. The dehydration occurs because our bodies use more water during an illness; lose water in urine, bowel actions and vomiting as well as by perspiration and breathing. The water in that urine or diarrhoea or vomit or perspiration was an essential part of the body tissues perhaps only an hour previously. Unless the water is replaced, the body cells become dehydrated and this can lead to death.

You can prevent or reduce dehydration by making certain that you or the person for whom you are caring takes sufficient fluid to replace that lost (see chart).

The sick person can take unlimited amounts of soups or broths but glucose containing drinks must be given only after consideration of the blood or urinary glucose levels. For instance, a person with a blood glucose level greater than 10 mmol/L or 2 per cent glucose in the urine would not be given normal Coca Cola but would be given Diet Coke. A blood glucose level less than 10 mmol/l or urine free of glucose however would require fruit juices or ordinary coca cola, lemonade etc.

Sick Days

EQUIVALENT CARBOHYDRATE EXCHANGES

USUAL FOOD

Bread or toast (1 slice)

Cereal – cornflakes or rice bubbles (¾ cup)

Rolled oats (¾ cup)
Saos (2)
Arrowroot biscuits (2)

Crumpets (½)
English muffins (½)

Boiled rice (⅓ cup)

Canned soups (¾ cup made up with water)

SICK DAYS

Sweetened jelly (½ – NOT low cal)

Ice cream (½ cup)
Custard with sugar (½ cup)

Honey (3 tsp)
Sugar (1 tablespoon)
Sweetened ice block (1 small or 90 ml)

Egg flip – sweetened (8 oz)

Tea or Coffee + 4 tsp sugar

Milk (10 oz)

Coke, lemonade or other sweetened soft drink (¾ cup – NOT low calorie)

Unsweetened tinned fruit (¾ cup)

Orange juice (¾ cup)
Apple juice (½ cup)
Pineapple juice (½ cup)

Orange (1 medium)
Banana (1 small)

Unflavoured yoghurt (300 g)
Flavoured (sweetened) yoghurt (100 g)

Vomiting

Home is not normally the place for a vomiting person with diabetes. A single vomit however is not necessarily a cause for alarm but repeated vomiting, particularly in a child or teenager, may be a prelude to diabetic ketoacidosis and medical attention must be obtained urgently. It is possible for the doctor to give an injection to stop vomiting but this should not be repeated in children as it can itself lead to other problems of a non-diabetic nature.

In Hospital

It is quite likely that the hospital does not have your particular insulin or that the ward does not have a glucose meter. Therefore bring your own insulin, syringes, glucose meter and blood strips with you to the hospital.

The staff in intensive care units, endocrine or diabetic wards are knowledgeable in the management of diabetes but this may not be true for some of the medical and nursing staff in other areas of a hospital. Carefully watch the technique of the staff undertaking your blood glucose readings or preferably do them yourself. Remember, however, your stay in hospital could be made unpleasant if your attitude to the staff is unnecessarily critical or antagonistic. Don't be afraid to ask questions and offer assistance.

❑ ❑ ❑

Sick Days

Summary

1. **Always take your normal insulin dosage or tablets even if you are too sick to eat.**
2. **Test blood and/or urine for glucose every four hours, or more often.**
3. **Test your urine for ketones.**
4. **Endeavour to consume your normal carbohydrate intake.**
5. **Fluid by mouth is essential.**

Medical attention is required if:

Vomiting persists
Ketones are present and particularly if they increase in concentration
The blood glucose gets higher
The sick person appears drowsy or confused
The method of giving additional insulin is not understood
The nature of the intercurrent illness is not known
Commonsense indicates the need

CHAPTER 14

Diabetes and Other Medications

By Clinical Professor Gillian Shenfield
Head of Dept. of Clinical Pharmacology
Royal North Shore Hospital
Sydney

Diabetes can occur at any age and is a life-long problem. It is therefore only to be expected that people with diabetes will, at various times, have other medical problems.

Everyone in the community gets coughs, colds and chest infections. Kidney and bladder infections are extremely common, and as we get older, more and more people get arthritis, high blood pressure, heart and circulation problems.

In diabetes, it is particularly important to control high blood pressure and many people with diabetes are on blood pressure lowering medicines. In fact someone with diabetes, somewhere in the world, is likely to be taking any of the tablets available on prescription or over-the-counter at the chemist or supermarket.

Some of these medications can affect diabetes in a variety of ways. This chapter cannot address all such possible interactions and will only consider common problems that may arise. It is important to realise that the "interactions" described here are those that may occur, they will not necessarily happen to everyone with diabetes who takes the tablets described.

To avoid problems it is essential that any doctor or pharmacist knows that you have diabetes and that you are obtaining medications for another condition. If in doubt ask for advice from an expert.

The medications to be discussed will be described by their "proper" or "generic" names. Where an individual drug is concerned its most common "trade name" is also included, eg. oats as a generic food are known under the trade names "Uncle Toby's Oats", "Mrs McWilliams Oats" etc.

One other important point about the effects that medications may have on diabetes relates to the time course of any interaction. In general the highest risk of a problem is when a medication is stopped or started or the dose is changed.

A new tablet for blood pressure, a change in dose of a tablet for arthritis or stopping a sulphonamide antibiotic may all cause problems. Long-term treatment with any other medication, together with a diabetes tablet, is unlikely to trouble you since a balance between them will have been achieved. Therefore be aware of change and take extra care with tests when a new medication is stopped or started.

There are a variety of ways in which medications may interact with diabetes and it is impossible to generalise. I will discuss some of the potential problems under separate headings.

Medications that may raise blood glucose

Table 1 lists some commonly used medications that may cause blood glucose to increase. It indicates the mechanism (where known) by which this is believed to occur and also shows whether it is likely to happen to people with diabetes on insulin, on tablets or on diet alone. The reason there are differences between the three groups is that sometimes the other medication has a direct effect on diabetes and sometimes it is interacting with the treatment for diabetes.

Various medications for children are made up as very sweet syrups and large volumes may cause blood glucose to rise. Diuretics which are used to treat blood pressure or ankle swelling can have a similar effect.

In some mild cases of Type 2 diabetes just stopping a diuretic may be sufficient to allow an individual to manage on diet alone, without any

TABLE 1

COMMON MEDICATIONS THAT MAY RAISE BLOOD GLUCOSE

LIKELY TO HAVE EFFECT WITH

MEDICATION	MECHANISM	INSULIN	TABLETS	DIET
Antibiotic syrups for children	Contain sugar	++	N/A	N/A
Antihistamine syrups for children	Contain sugar	++	N/A	N/A
Corticosteroids	Oppose insulin action	++	++	++
Cough mixtures in syrup	Contain sugar	++	++	++
Diuretics	Block insulin secretion	±	++	++
Nifedipine (Adalat)	Delays insulin action	±	+	+
Oral contraceptives	Oppose insulin action	+	N/A	N/A
Phenytoin (Dilantin)	Blocks insulin secretion	±	+	+
Phenothiazine Tranquilisers	?	+	+	+

N/A Not applicable

tablets to control the blood glucose.

Phenytoin (Dilantin) used to treat epilepsy, is a good example of a situation where a medication is taken over a very long period and problems are only likely to arise if phenytoin is stopped, started or changed in dose.

Oral contraceptive pills are not contraindicated in diabetes but are most likely to be used in women taking insulin. They may increase blood glucose slightly and hence the insulin dose may need to be increased, but in many women blood glucose control is more stable over a menstrual cycle when a contraceptive pill is taken.

Medications that may lower blood glucose

Table 2 is in the same format as table 1 and indicates those medications most likely to lower blood glucose. In this case you will see that most of the problems arise in those individuals who are taking tablets (usually the sulphonylureas) to treat their diabetes.

The reason for this is that many medications raise the amount of sulphonylurea in the blood and hence increase their effect.

This occurs either by reducing the rate at which sulphonylureas are removed from the body or by displacing them from the carrier proteins to which they are usually attached in the blood. This

TABLE 2
COMMON MEDICATIONS THAT MAY LOWER BLOOD GLUCOSE

LIKELY TO HAVE EFFECT WITH

MEDICATION	MECHANISM	INSULIN	TABLETS	DIET
Alcohol	Stops liver producing glucose	++	++	±
Allopurinol (Zyloprim)	Increases amount of Sulphonylurea in blood	–	+	–
Angiotensin Converting Enzyme inhibitors	Increase insulin action	+	+	–
Aspirin	Increases amount of sulphonylurea in blood	–	++	–
Beta–blocking medications	Oppose action of Adrenaline	++	+	–
Clofibrate (Atromid–S)	?	±	++	–
Monoamine oxidase antidepressants	Interfere with adrenaline action	++	++	–
Non–steroidal anti–inflammatory medications	Increase amount of sulphonylurea in blood	–	++	–
Oxytetracycline	Slows insulin removal	++	+	–
Sulphonamide antibiotics	Increase amount of sulphonylurea in blood	–	++	–
Warfarin	Increase amount of sulphonyurea in blood	–	++	–

type of interaction is obviously not going to occur on patients on insulin or diet only.

Blood glucose is most unlikely to fall as a result of another medication in anyone treated with diet alone.

Alcohol, although not strictly a medication, has been included because it is so important. In moderation it is unlikely to cause hypoglycaemia but if taken without food or in large quantities it can lower blood glucose in anyone with diabetes irrespective of treatment.

Angiotensin converting enzyme inhibitors (Accupril, Amprace, Asig, Capoten, Coversyl, Monopril, Prinivil, Ramace, Renitec) and beta-blocking drugs (many different ones) may be used to treat high blood pressure or heart disease. Their actions are very different but they can all decrease blood glucose and cause a need for a decreased dose of insulin or tablets.

Diabetes and Other Medications

Clofibrate (Atromid-S) is used to lower cholesterol and allopurinol (Zyloprim) to treat gout. "Non-steroidal inflammatory drugs" refers to all the medications prescribed to relieve pain in arthritis.

In some instances, if you are given one of these medications, no change will be seen in blood glucose but some people are particularly susceptible to interactions and may need a changed dose of insulin or diabetes tablets.

The most common examples of sulphonamide containing antibiotics, which can produce low blood glucose, are Septrin and Bactrim and these can be a problem to people taking sulphonylurea tablets. Sudden drops in blood glucose can occur one or two days after starting the antibiotics.

Other antibiotics (except for oxytetracycline) do not cause this effect, but, of course, blood glucose may fall as the infection comes under control.

Medications that alter response to glucose or insulin

The beta-blocking medications block some of the actions of the naturally occurring hormones adrenaline and noradrenaline. These act in the body to oppose insulin effects and, if they themselves are rendered less active, insulin will have a greater than normal effect.

This causes a reduction in blood glucose but also has other results.

Many of the symptoms of hypoglycaemia — the "warning signs" such as sweating, fast pulse and anxiety, — are due to the actions of adrenaline.

In the presence of beta-blockers these signs and symptoms are lost and blood glucose can drop considerably without the warning that gives you time to take some form of sugar.

In addition, adrenaline is one of the substances that helps blood glucose to recover, after a hypoglycaemic episode, in insulin dependent diabetes.

If the action of adrenaline is blocked this recovery can be considerably delayed. Beta-blockers should therefore always be used with caution in people with diabetes, especially those on insulin. Some of the newer beta-blocking agents e.g. atenolol (Noten, Tenormin) and metoprolol (Betaloc, Lopressor) have a so called "selective" action and only oppose some of the effects of adrenaline. They are therefore less likely to cause many of the above problems.

Cigarettes are usually not considered to be medications but they are certainly drugs in the sense of highly active foreign substances that enter the body and affect its functions. Smoking is not recommended for anyone, particularly anyone with diabetes, since it can increase the risk of abnormalities in the heart and circulation.

In addition it has been found that, in Type 1 diabetes there is a reduced rate of absorption of insulin in the first 30 minutes after smoking. Diabetic smokers need, on average, 15-20 per cent more insulin than non-smokers and heavy smokers may need 30 per cent more. Any change in smoking habits could therefore produce alterations in how much insulin gets into the blood stream.

If a heavy smoker suddenly gives up the habit, up to 30 per cent more insulin could be absorbed and blood glucose could drop. This is not a reason to keep on smoking but indicates a need for care when changing long entrenched habits.

Medications which can affect urine glucose tests

There are two main ways of testing for glucose in the urine. The first uses the general chemical reaction known as "a reducing reaction" and chemical test tablets work in this way.

They are used less these days but they do give an accurate quantitative measure of how much glucose is in the urine. A series of other chemicals can also act as "reducing substances" and can therefore give false positive tests, i.e. the urine appears to contain glucose when it does not really do so. Medications likely to do this are listed in table 3.

The second sort of test uses a more specific glucose oxidase enzyme to provide a very accurate qualitative and semi-quantitative measure of glucose in the urine.

All the sticks available in Australia (including Testape) work in this way. It is very

Diabetes and Other Medications

TABLE 3
MEDICATIONS THAT MAY INTERFERE WITH URINE TESTS

Medications (Generic Name)	Clinitest Tablets	Stick and Tape Tests
Ascorbic Acid (Vitamin C)	+	–
Cephalosporins	+	0
Chloral Hydrate	? +	0
Isoniazid	+	0
Levodopa	+	–
Methyldopa	+	0
Nalidixic Acid	+	0
Probenecid	+	0
Salicylicates (Aspirin)	+	0
Sulphonamides	? +	0
Tetracyclines	? +	
Nitrofurantoin	? +	0
Phenazopyridine (Pyridium)	0	– sticks +Testape

Key
- – False negative
- + False Positive
- 0 No known effect
- ? Possible effect (not fullly proven)

unusual to get false positive results with these sticks but it is possible to get false negatives, i.e. the stick says no glucose is present when in reality it is present.

This is caused by break-down products of drugs inhibiting the glucose oxidase reaction. Somewhat paradoxically ascorbic acid (Vitamin C) interferes with both forms of test, but in opposite directions.

For this reason, some testing sticks include a patch to measure ascorbic acid i.e. if it is found to be present in the urine a negative glucose result must be interpreted with caution.

If you are taking one of the medications on the list for any length of time it will be necessary to get blood glucose tested in order to check accuracy of your urine readings.

Unusual interactions

In addition to the effects above, alcohol can interact with some of the sulphonylurea tablets (especially chlorpropamide and tolbutamide) and cause flushing. This is an unpleasant effect in which the face becomes hot and red. It may be associated with nausea. If you only drink alcohol occasionally then the problem is of no

Diabetes and Other Medications

significance, certainly no permanent harm is caused. If you are a regular drinker and flushing occurs, it is probably best to ask your doctor to change you over to another tablet.

Interactions with complications of diabetes

The many possible complications of diabetes are described elsewhere in this book. Some of them, such as heart disease, may need treatment with special medications. In some cases care is needed to avoid substances that may make a problem worse or confuse the process of diagnosis.

Thus if someone with diabetes has impotence, before this can definitely be attributed to the diabetes, it is important to make sure that they are not taking blood pressure treatments that may also cause impotence e.g. methyldopa (Aldomet), beta-blocking medications etc.

If you have autonomic neuropathy this can produce a low blood pressure and it is important to avoid other medications that can also have an effect in lowering blood pressure e.g. angina treatments such as isosorbide (Isordil, Isotrate), nifedipine (Adalat), felodipine (Agon, Plendil). If you have any problems with low blood pressure, nitrate patches and ointments (Nitro-bid, Nitrodisc, Transiderm nitro) should only be used after full discussion with your doctor.

Sometimes diabetes can impair the circulation to the hands and feet making them cold and very numb. In this situation medications that can also reduce the circulation e.g. beta-blockers, ergot containing migraine tablets, should be avoided.

❏ ❏ ❏

Conclusions

This is not a complete list but should give you some indication of the difficulties that may occur with medications and diabetes.

Diabetes involves the whole body and it is therefore necessary to think about the whole system when using any other medication. The medication rules are:

- **Always make sure that any doctor or pharmacist you see knows that you have diabetes and knows what treatment you are taking.**
- **Never take a new medication without making sure that you know if it may affect your diabetes and, if so, what precautions you should take.**
- **Realise that problems are most likely to occur at times of dose change or stopping or starting medications. At these times take extra care.**

DIABETES & YOU
An owner's manual

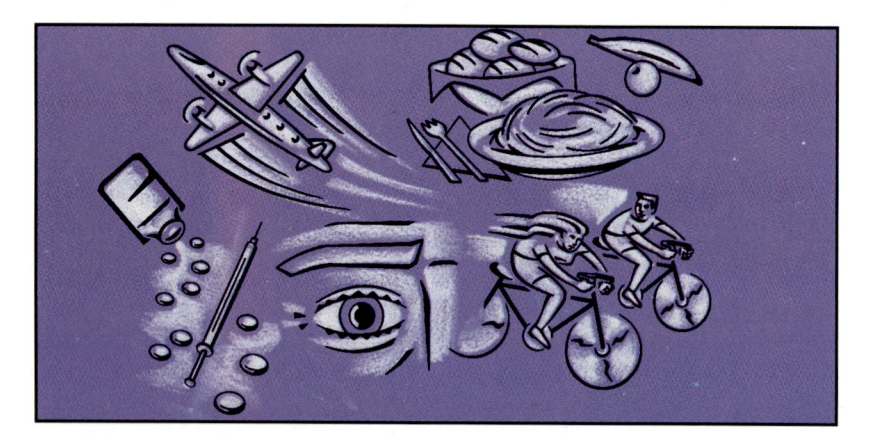

COMPLICATIONS

❑ **Chronic Complications of Diabetes**

Important factors
Eye damage
Blood vessel blockage
Kidney damage
Infections
Nerve damage
Sudden hypos
How to reduce chances of complications
Minor complications

❑ **Diabetes and Eyes**

The chances of retinopathy
Effects of diabetes on vision
Who should examine
When examinations should be carried out
Testing for retinopathy
The control of diabetes and retinopathy

❑ **Caring for Feet**

Nerve damage and damage to blood vessels
Footwear
Footcare
Things to avoid
Foot first aid

❑ **Diabetes and Pregnancy**

Metabolic changes during pregnancy
Pregnancy in women with pre-existing diabetes
Common concerns about pregnancy and the baby
Presence of complications in the mother
Planned pregnancy
Diabetes developing during pregnancy

❑ **Diabetes and Female Sexuality**

Emotional factors
High blood glucose levels
Sexual counselling

❑ **Sexual Problems in Men**

Impotence
Treatment
Penile injection
Penile implant
Vacuum device

❑ **You and Your Health Care Team**

Your responsibilities
Your doctor's responsibilities
Keeping track of your care
Health care professionals

CHAPTER 15

Chronic Complications of Diabetes

By Dr Warren Kidson
Visiting Endocrinologist
Prince of Wales and Prince of Wales Children's Hospital
Visiting Physician in Diabetes
Hornsby and Kuringai Hospital, Sydney

The word "chronic" suggests that the problem develops after many years of diabetes or, alternatively, that it is present for many years once it develops. Some of these complications however can develop after only six or twelve months of high blood glucose. What are the complications of diabetes and what are the factors that cause them?

Important Factors

A list of those factors that are known to be important in causing complications is set out below.

It should also be remembered that some people inherit from their family a protection from some of the complications of diabetes while other people inherit an increased susceptibility. One's individual susceptibility to complications however cannot be determined.

High blood glucose is the most important factor in the cause of long-term diabetic complications. High blood glucose acts by attaching itself to different protein molecules throughout the body causing damage to the clotting factors in the blood and toughening or ageing of the "strengthening" fibres in the large and small blood vessels and in the joints. High blood glucose, along with a deficiency of insulin, can cause a build up of poisons in the eye and in the nerves. High blood fats, high cholesterol and overweight tend to accelerate the build up of cholesterol and other deposits on the lining of blood vessels, accelerating their blockage. The blockage of these blood vessels is also greatly accelerated by untreated high blood pressure which can also damage the eyes and kidneys.

The second single most important factor in

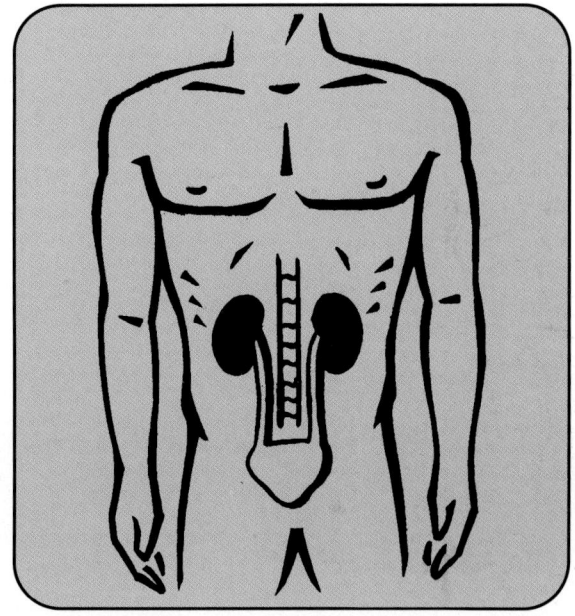

The kidneys are organs that can be affected by diabetes.

the development of complications in the eyes, kidneys and blood vessels, particularly in the blood vessels of the legs, is tobacco smoking. It is vitally important that people with diabetes avoid cigarettes.

An excess of alcohol can aggravate nerve damage whilst physical fitness is thought to protect the body from blood vessel blockage and possibly from eye damage.

Eye damage (Retinopathy and Cataract)

These complications in the eye are described elsewhere in the book (Chapter 16, Diabetes and Eyes). It is important that the person with diabetes has regular eye checks from his diabetes specialist or his medical eye specialist (ophthalmologist).

Chronic Complications of Diabetes

Blood Vessel Blockage (Vascular Disease)

Blood vessel blockage in the legs, heart or brain can occur in people without diabetes but, unfortunately, it occurs far more commonly in people with diabetes.

BLOOD VESSEL BLOCKAGE IN THE HEART (ISCHAEMIC HEART DISEASE)

This is caused by progressive narrowing of the coronary arteries which nourish the heart muscle. As the lining of the blood vessel thickens, the flow of blood is impeded and the heart muscle is deprived of oxygen and nourishment.

Symptoms are intermittent chest pain, generally brought on by exertion, and relieved after a few minutes by rest. This is due to a partial blockage and is known as angina.

Quite often the person with diabetes is unaware that he has narrowed blood vessels in the heart until they block completely, causing a coronary occlusion or heart attack.

The usual symptom of a heart attack is a heavy pressing pain across the chest, sometimes going into the neck or down the left arm. Unlike the intermittent pains of angina, the pain may last several hours and usually comes on when the patient is resting.

Provided the area of heart muscle affected is not large, healing usually takes place and the patient is able to get back to normal activity. Diseased heart arteries can sometimes be bypassed surgically.

BLOOD VESSEL BLOCKAGE TO THE BRAIN (CEREBROVASCULAR DISEASE)

A blockage of an artery in or leading to the brain can lead to a "stroke" or cerebrovascular accident where the symptoms are usually those of loss of speech, paralysis down one side of the body, loss of vision, coma or confusion.

Rehabilitation including physiotherapy and speech therapy can often allow the stroke

FACTORS	COMPLICATIONS OF DIABETES				
responsible for damage	Blood vessel blockage in heart, brain & legs	Eye damage	Kidney damage	Infections of vagina, bladder & kidneys	Nerve damage
High blood glucose levels	+	+++	++	+++	+++
High blood pressure	+++	++	++	–	–
Tobacco smoking	+++	++	+	–	–
High blood fats and cholesterol	+++	–	–	–	–
Excess alcohol	–	–	–	–	++
Lack of exercise	++	+	–	–	–
Overweight	++	+	–	–	–
Duration of diabetes	++	+	+	–	+

Chronic Complications of Diabetes

sufferer to return to an active life.

Symptoms such as temporary loss of speech, temporary paralysis, temporary impairment of vision, confusion or convulsions can be due to a partial blockage of a blood vessel into the brain. This situation needs urgent medical attention because anti-clotting treatment or surgery to clean out the arteries in the neck can prevent a subsequent stroke.

BLOOD VESSEL BLOCKAGE IN THE LEGS (PERIPHERAL VASCULAR DISEASE)

Symptoms are generally pain in one or both calf muscles during or after walking. Later, ulcers of the toes and feet may appear. Chronic pain can be felt in the feet at night.

Occasionally blood vessels may be cleaned out, or by-passed, by surgery. Generally, however, in diabetes the tendency is for the blockage to occur in blood vessels that are so small that surgery is not possible.

If the blockage is very severe, gangrene may develop in the toes and feet, necessitating surgical treatment, usually amputation of the foot and leg below the knee.

It is important to examine your feet from time to time to look for ulcers or infection. Your doctor will test the pulses in your feet and legs occasionally.

Kidney Damage (Nephropathy)

Diabetic kidney damage is usually due to changes in the small blood vessels leading to the filtering system of the kidney or to the smaller blood vessels within the filtering system itself. It is a completely painless process and cannot be detected even by a physical examination by a doctor.

Detection of nephropathy however is possible by pathology testing of the urine for protein, of the blood for urea and of the blood and urine for creatinine.

Infections of the Vagina, Bladder and Kidney

People with diabetes have a higher chance of developing infections in the vagina, bladder and kidneys than people without diabetes.

The vaginal secretions and urine of people with diabetes often contain increased amounts of glucose, providing an excellent source of food on which germs (bacteria and fungi) can grow.

If the nerves to the bladder have been damaged by diabetes, the bladder may not empty completely when passing urine, leaving some urine within the bladder in which germs may multiply.

Symptoms of vaginal infection are itching of the vagina and vulval areas, often associated with a discharge from the vagina onto the pants. This can be treated by pessaries and creams. Occasionally a course of tablets taken by mouth by both the patient and her sexual partner is also needed. Lowering high blood glucose levels to normal often helps the treatment.

Symptoms of bladder and kidney infections are the passing of small amounts of urine at more frequent intervals both by day and by night and a burning discomfort or pain while passing urine. Backache is also an occasional symptom of kidney infection.

Infection of the bladder is called cystitis whilst infection of the kidney is called pyelitis or pyelonephritis, but both infections usually occur together. These infections are diagnosed by a microscope examination of a specimen of urine and by a urine culture test. Infections are usually treated effectively by antibiotics taken by mouth.

Prompt treatment of bladder and kidney infections is important as these infections, if allowed to continue, may result in chronic kidney damage.

Nerve Damage (Neuropathy)

Nerve damage can be caused by high blood glucose levels and excessive alcohol consumption.

Nerve damage in the legs causes numbness, coldness of the legs, tingling, pins and needles sensation in the feet and burning pains in the legs and feet, usually more noticeable in bed at night.

Numbness, tingling and pins and needles sensation in the hands is more often due to compression of a nerve as it runs through a bony tunnel in the wrist, a condition which can be relieved by a simple operation. This is relatively common in people with diabetes.

Chronic Complications of Diabetes

If the nerve damage extends to the nerves in the tummy and chest, the most common symptom is that of sexual impotence in men, that is the inability to achieve an erection of the penis at the time of sexual intercourse. Impotence can also be due to blockage of the blood vessels supplying the penis with blood (Chapter 20, Sexual Problems in Men).

Nerve damage in the tummy can also cause paralysis of the valve at the bottom of the stomach which can lead to vomiting or the collection of two or three meals in the stomach before opening of the stomach valve, leading to marked swings in blood glucose levels from low levels to high levels. This condition can be treated with medication such as metoclopramide or cisapride.

Very rarely nerve damage in the tummy can lead to intermittent diarrhoea, particularly at night, and faintness or dizziness on standing up out of a bed or chair. Nerve damage in the tummy can lead to incomplete bladder emptying Nerve damage is detected by testing for different types of sensation in the feet and legs and by testing the knee and ankle reflexes.

Nerve damage can lead to loss of sensation in the feet which allows the person with diabetes to damage their feet because they cannot feel pain. This can lead to ulcers on the bottom of the feet which can penetrate into the bone leading to osteomyelitis, a chronic infection in the bones which may lead to the need for amputation if not treated vigorously from the earliest time of infection or ulceration.

It is very important for people with diabetes to examine their feet at least every second or third day.

Sudden, severe hypos without warning (Hypoglycaemic Unawareness)

Type 1 diabetes is due to an attack by the immune system on the insulin cells of the pancreas gland. Unfortunately the immune system often does not stop its attack at the insulin cells of the pancreas gland but often goes on to attack other glands and tissues in the body.

The damage in diabetes often goes on to affect the cells in the pancreas gland that secrete the hormone glucagon and the central core of the adrenal glands that secretes adrenalin. Both glucagon and adrenalin are important in protection from hypoglycaemia because they switch on glucose production in the liver at times of hypoglycaemia. Adrenalin is doubly important because the secretion of increased amounts of adrenalin at the time of hypoglycaemia also causes the symptoms of shaking, sweating and palpitations, the early warning symptoms of hypoglycaemia. Adrenalin secretion may also be lost by damage to the nerves in the tummy.

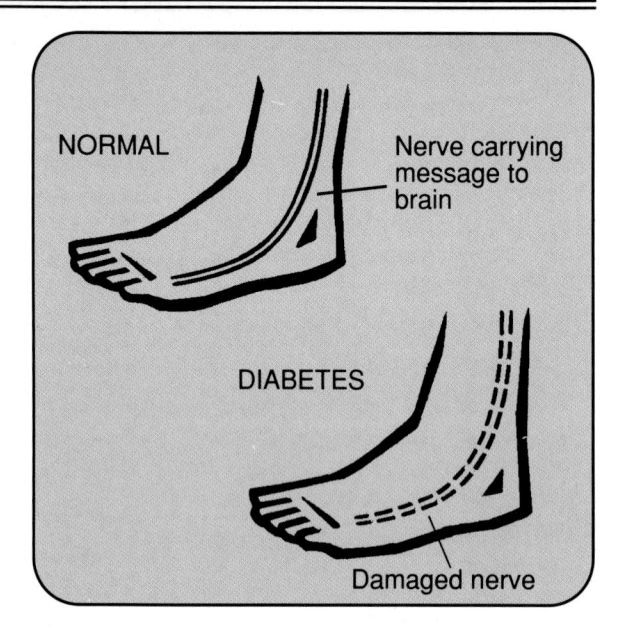

Therefore, if diabetes destroys ones' ability to secrete glucagon and adrenalin, hypos can occur without warning and can be even more severe.

How can you reduce your chances of the long-term complications of diabetes?

1. Attempt to keep blood glucose levels, both after meals as well as before meals, in the range of 3-8mmol/L and certainly no higher than 11mmol/l on most tests. A few weeks of high blood glucose levels is unlikely to do very much long-term harm.

2. At all costs do not smoke.

3. Have regular physical exercise, keep your weight down to your so-called "ideal body

weight" and keep your blood fats and cholesterol down.
4. If your blood pressure is high have your doctor treat it.
5. Have your eyes checked regularly by a medical eye specialist (ophthalmologist) or your diabetes specialist. Examine your feet regularly and get your doctor to check your feet for blood vessel blockage, nerve damage, ulcers, ingrown toe-nails and tinea from time to time.
6. Your blood pressure should be checked regularly and you should have occasional pathology tests to check your cholesterol, blood fats, kidney function and average blood sugar control.

The number of complications caused by diabetes has diminished greatly over the past 10 to 15 years because of the knowledge that has been gained during that time.

Minor complications of diabetes

Hollows in the fat tissue (Fat Atrophy)

Fat atrophy is the loss of fat between the skin and muscle at injection sites. It is probably due to an individual reaction to certain types of insulin by the fat tissue and is now extremely rare since the introduction of highly purified insulins and since the introduction of human insulins.

Lumps of fatty tissue (Fat Hypertrophy)

Fat hypertrophy – the opposite of fat atrophy, also occurs at injection sites and consists of an increase or accumulation of fat between the skin and muscle and probably the result of injections being given too often in one place. The cure is to avoid giving injections in the areas of hypertrophy and to rotate injection sites over a far greater area of body than previously used. If you are using the tummy, the whole area, the front and the sides, should be used.

Insulin Allergy

Insulin allergy consists of redness, pain or itching, generally at the injection sites although the itching may occur over the entire body. This complication usually develops in the first month or two on insulin and disappears within six to eight weeks. It is now extremely rare since the introduction of highly purified insulin and since the introduction of human insulins.

Necrobiosis Lipoidica Diabeticorum

This is a rare condition involving the tissues beneath the skin and accompanied by thinning of the skin, usually at the front or side part of the leg between the knee and ankle. It does not appear to be related to diabetic control and is very difficult to treat. It may come on after many years of diabetes but occasionally may develop many years before diabetes develops.

Swelling of the ankles and face (Insulin Oedema)

This problem consists of swelling of the ankles and occasionally the face and hands because of fluid retention. It usually only occurs after the blood sugars have been very high for several months and after the blood sugar has been brought down at the start of insulin treatment or after an increase in the insulin dose. The cause of this condition is not known. It usually gets better by itself but occasionally anti-fluid tablets, (diuretics), are needed.

Xanthoma and Xanthelasma

These conditions are due to excess cholesterol or fats accumulating in the skin. They usually consist of red or yellowish spots around the elbows and knees or occasionally in the palms of the hands or on the chest or below the eyelids.

They may indicate poor blood sugar control, excessive fat in the blood or excess alcohol consumption.

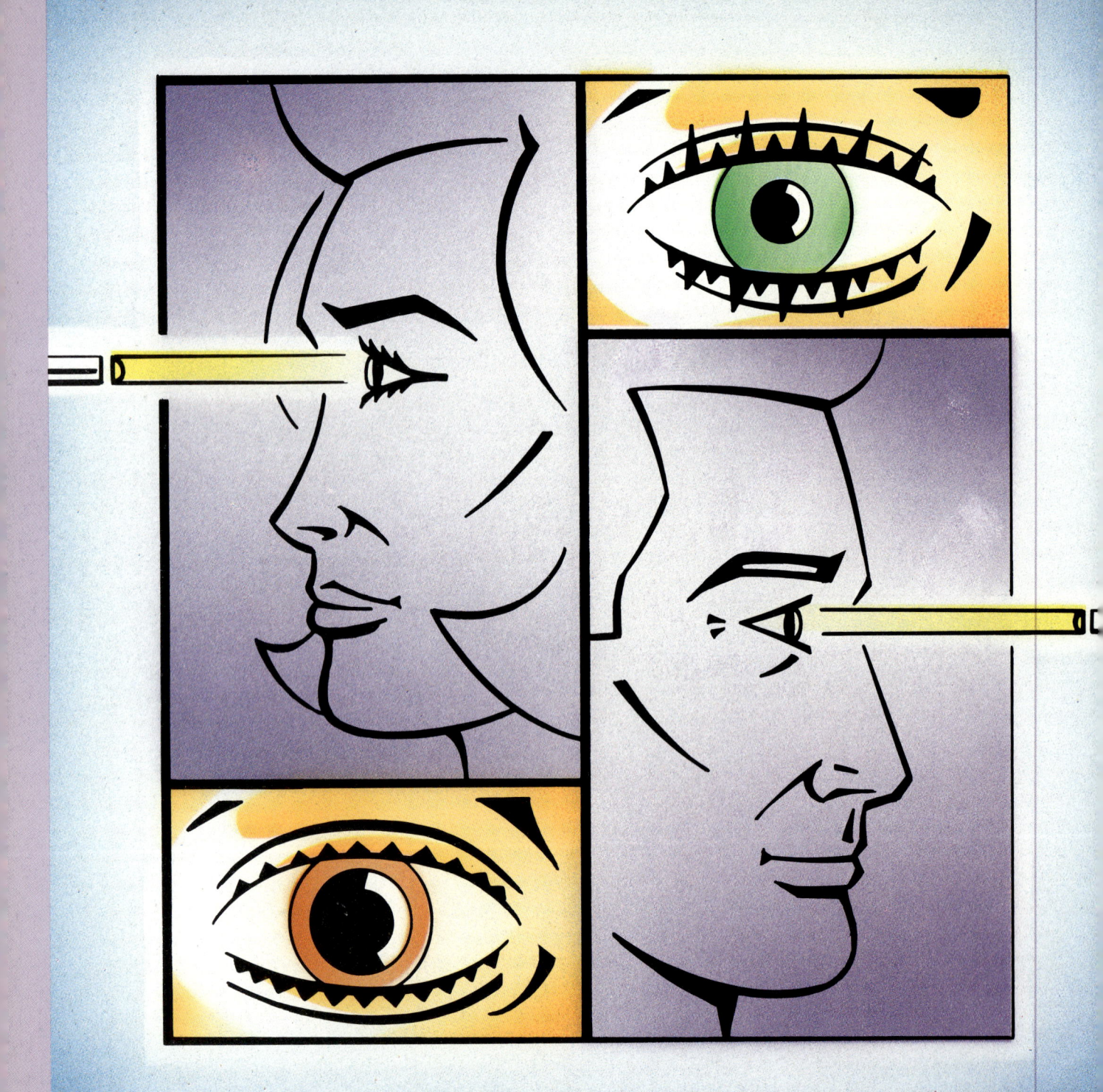

CHAPTER 16

Diabetes and Eyes

By Assoc. Prof. Paul Mitchell
University of Sydney Eye Clinic
Westmead Hospital

Eye damage is a common "complication" of diabetes but happily, through better prevention and treatment it is becoming a less common cause of blindness in Australia and overseas.

The good news is that statistics show blindness caused by diabetes is on the decrease. Figures compiled in Newcastle show that diabetic retinopathy was the cause of blindness in 7 per cent of people registered for the blind pension during the last ten years, compared with almost 12 per cent for the previous 15 year period. In the latest UK figures (1986) diabetic retinopathy as a cause of blindness was down to 3 per cent of the total.

While these figures are encouraging, ophthalmologists (medically qualified eye doctors) in Australia still see many diabetic patients losing vision- in most cases unnecessarily.

There are a number of reasons for this.

Firstly, many people with diabetes and their doctors may not strive for low enough blood glucose levels and seem satisfied with what we now believe is less than adequate control.

This attitude is particularly common in people with older-onset diabetes, that is, diagnosed after age 30. Too often people believe Type 2 diabetes is "just a touch of sugar". This is not the case and some people with older-onset or Type 2 diabetes actually achieve better control and feel better, on insulin.

Secondly, many people with diabetes do not attend ophthalmologists for regular eye checks until after their vision has started to fail. Tragically, some older people do not visit an ophthalmologist until their second eye has become affected and vision has failed in both.

While ophthalmologists can help people affected by retinopathy, this is not the best time to start treatment. The ideal situation is to detect the earliest stages of retinopathy before there has been any effect on vision, and monitor its progress carefully. This enables the eye doctor to liaise closely with the person's diabetes doctor especially if the early eye damage is occurring faster than the length of time the person has had diabetes would suggest. It might also prompt them to look for other factors which could be important, like high blood pressure.

The chances of retinopathy

Retinopathy is very common in people with diabetes and is related strongly to the length of time diabetes has been present.

In all studies carried out in Australia so far, about one in three people with known diabetes has some evidence of retinopathy and of these, another one in three has retinopathy which has either damaged vision or threatens to. After five years of diabetes about 20 per cent of people have some signs of retinopathy while after ten years, around 50 per cent, or one in two has some retinopathy present, although this does not mean all are at risk of losing sight.

Retinopathy which damages or threatens to damage vision takes longer to develop but is seen in about 15 to 20 per cent of people after ten years and about a third of people after 20 years of diabetes. While the risk seems slightly higher for people on insulin, it is still very substantial in people treated by diet or tablets.

The development of some retinopathy may therefore seem almost inevitable after a long duration of diabetes but the effect on vision is mostly preventable or can be decreased considerably with treatment.

Diabetes and Eyes

Effects of diabetes on vision

There are three ways diabetes can affect vision.

Retinopathy causes damage to the small blood vessels in the back of the eyes and may result in loss of vision due to obstruction, leak or haemorrhage.

The most severe loss of vision comes from *Proliferative Retinopathy* in which abnormal blood vessels grow from the optic nerve or other vessels because large areas of the eyes' circulation have been blocked by the diabetic process.

These "new" vessels are not helpful and tend to bleed and scar. While occurring in all age groups, this is commonest with Type 1 diabetes which has usually been present for a long time, often more than 20 years.

The most frequent cause is Maculopathy in which a leak occurs from blood vessels near the eye's centre of vision, leading to swelling and slow loss of reading vision. Maculopathy can occur in all age groups but is more common in people with Type 2 diabetes.

Finally, there is *Cataract*, an opacity, or opaqueness, which forms in the lens of the eye and is a common cause of decreased vision. Cataracts tend to develop earlier in people with diabetes, but they can be removed surgically with a lens implant. This is done exactly the same way as for people without diabetes, and usually with good results.

Who should examine

The examination should normally be done by an ophthalmologist but your diabetes doctor may also be able to check your vision and screen your retinae carefully after dilating your pupils with drops.

It is important that pupils are dilated with eye drops as it is only in this way that a good view of the retina can be achieved by the examiner.

When examinations should be carried out

Significant retinopathy threatening vision may be present in many people with diabetes before any effect on vision. In view of this and the beneficial effect of early laser treatment for vision-threatening retinopathy, regular retinal screening of all people with diabetes is recommended.

- For people with diabetes diagnosed before age 30, retinal examinations should start no later than after five years of diabetes and generally from age 10 onwards.
- For diabetes diagnosed at or after age 30, the examination should be made at the time of diabetes diagnosis, to detect any significant eye damage at that time.
- For both groups a subsequent examination is recommended every two years if no signs of retinopathy are found, and once any lesions are detected, a review is needed every 12 months or earlier.

There are some high risk groups – people with high blood pressure, kidney damage or poor diabetic control, who may need closer follow up. Retinopathy can progress through a pregnancy, so it is recommended that women with diabetes are examined prior to commencing a pregnancy, and followed through it if there are any signs detected.

If retinopathy is found shortly after the diagnosis of diabetes – usually in Type 2 diabetes, it can progress more rapidly despite good control and therefore close review is needed.

Of course if people with diabetes notice any change in vision they should see an eye doctor immediately.

Testing for retinopathy

Your eye doctor or his staff will test your distance vision carefully, with glasses if you wear them, and may either change the lens or use a pinhole to obtain the best vision. He may also check your eye pressures, as raised eye pressure or glaucoma is seen more commonly in people with diabetes. Your pupils will then be dilated with drops, a process which often takes half an hour to an hour.

Once pupils are dilated, the doctor will use an ophthalmoscope or other instruments with fairly bright lights to screen your retina for any signs of diabetic retinopathy. While mildly unpleasant, this examination only lasts a few minutes.

Diabetes and Eyes

If there is some evidence of eye damage, the doctor may recommend a test known as a fluorescein angiogram. In this test, dye is injected through a vein in the arm and a series of photographs taken as the dye passes through the blood vessels in the body and eyes.

Dye can be seen in the vessels of the retina and will show up the damaged areas in greater detail.

This test is usually only carried out when significant retinopathy is present. Nausea occurs in about one in four people. One interesting effect is that the skin remains yellow for a few hours, and urine for a day afterwards, as dye is passed out of the body.

Action if retinopathy threatens vision

If the eye doctor finds signs of proliferative retinopathy or maculopathy or if these stages appear to be imminent, he will probably recommend laser treatment.

This treatment has proven effective in many major trials and is now routine in all centres in Australia. It is an outpatient or rooms procedure and usually takes about 15 to 30 minutes per session.

Laser treatment for maculopathy is usually not painful, though for proliferative retinopathy large areas of the retina need treatment and this can be painful. A local anaesthetic through the lower eyelid – not into the eye, may be suggested

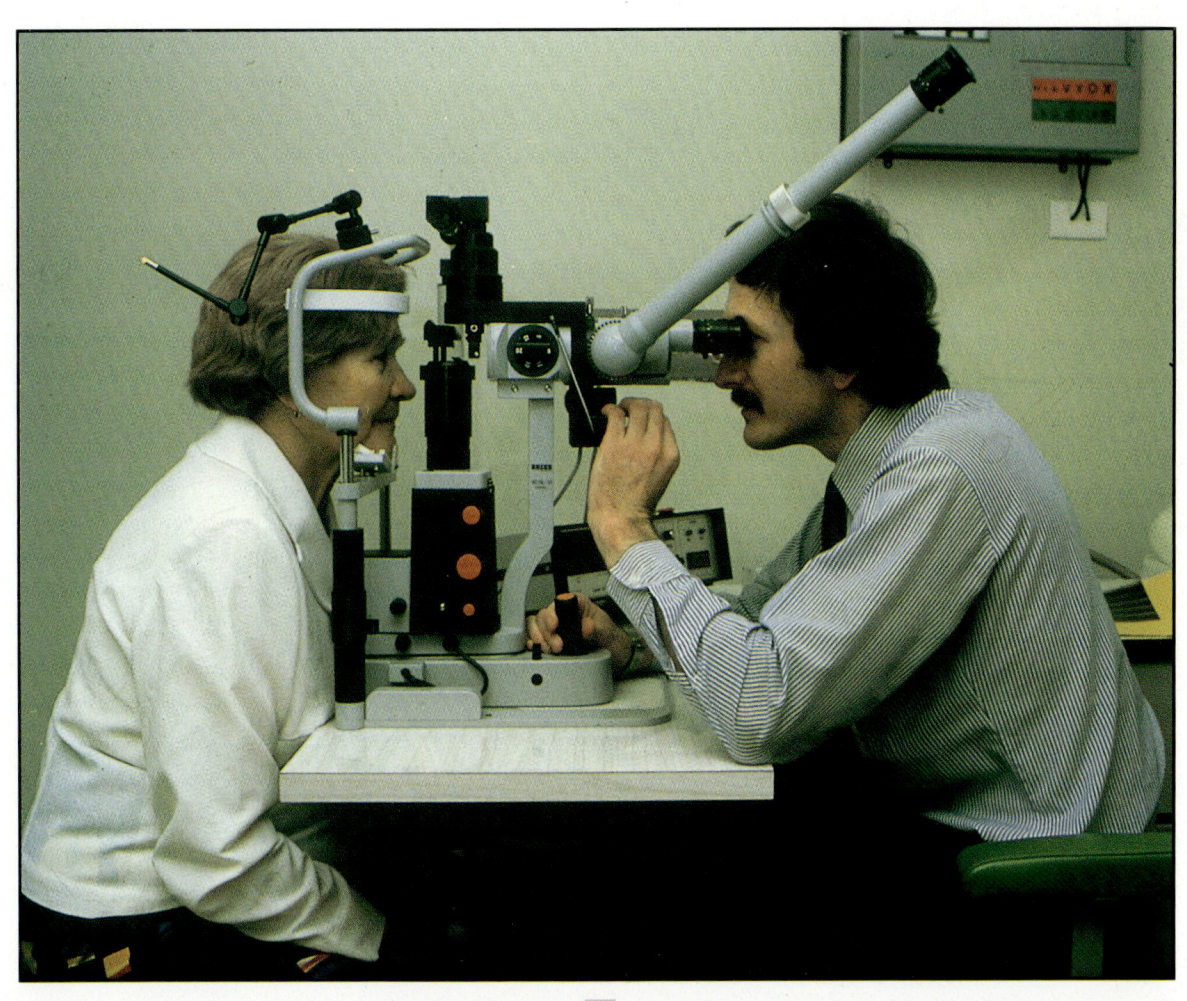

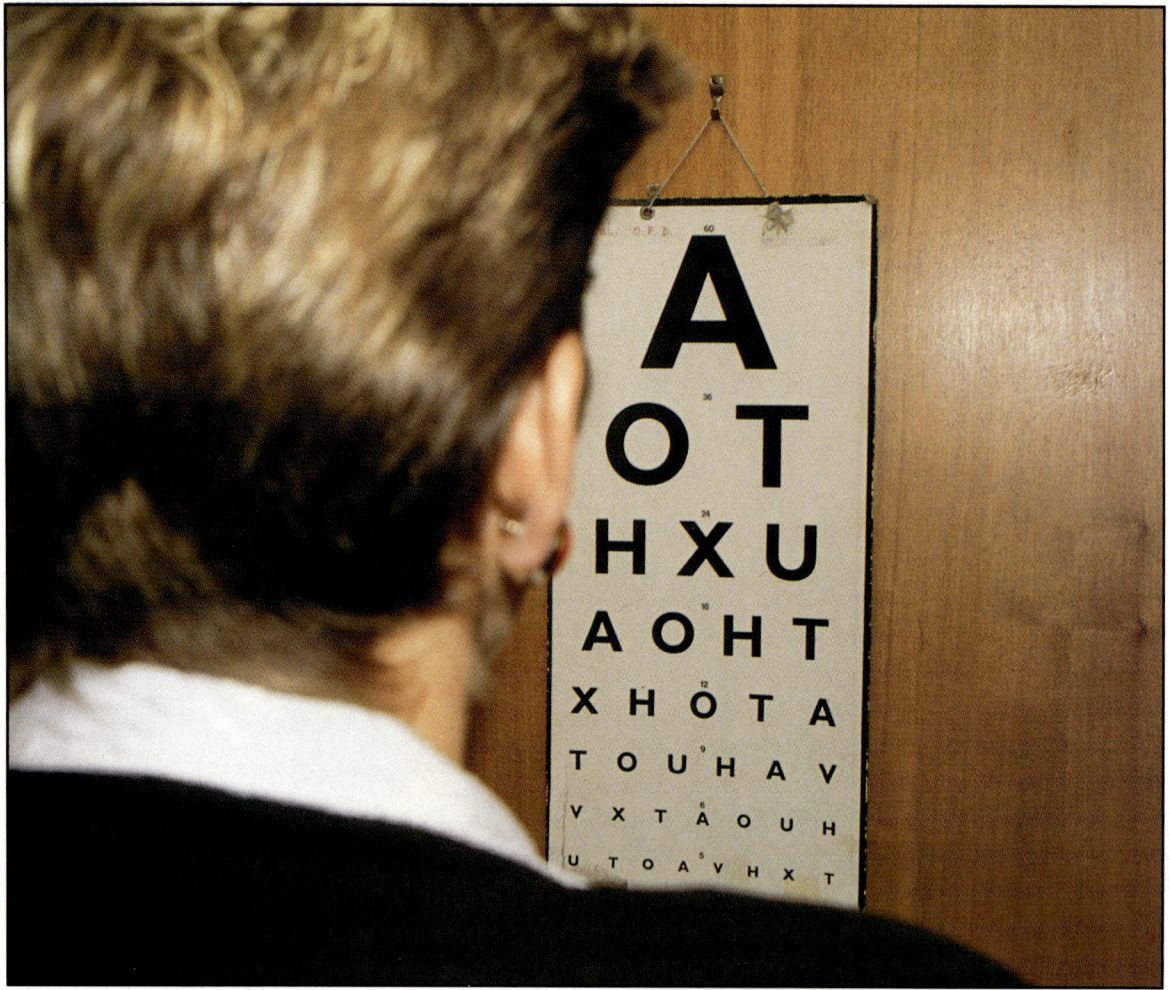

Your eyes can be tested by your ability to read a simple chart.

to prevent the pain, although many people seem to cope well without it.

A number of treatments may be required over a few weeks and vision may be blurred for a period.

The control of diabetes and retinopathy

There is increasing evidence that poor diabetic control increases the risk of retinopathy and its progression.

Further trials are underway to look at the relationship but in the meantime, it is best for people with diabetes to strive for as tight control as possible.

Once severe retinopathy has occurred, good control may not influence its course significantly. This is presumably because the changes which have occurred in the retina are already too advanced and to some extent are independent of the diabetes. If improved control does have a beneficial effect, this will probably be a few years down the track.

This emphasises the need to control diabetes as well as possible in the first few years, before any complications such as retinopathy have occurred. It also helps to explain why retinopathy continues to progress despite insulin treatment in people found to have retinopathy at the time of diagnosis.

Diabetes and Eyes

No medications have been found conclusively to be helpful in preventing or delaying retinopathy. Studies are currently underway to look at the possibility of a medication which may slow down the progression of retinopathy. Certainly people with high blood pressure seem to have an increased risk of retinopathy and so this must be treated as it could well delay or prevent retinopathy.

We should now be able to prevent much of the visual loss from diabetic retinopathy and as with all areas of diabetic control, education is important.

❑ ❑ ❑

Education of people with diabetes, their doctors and the general public are important steps in the battle to prevent diabetic blindness – a battle that happily, we appear to be winning.

CHAPTER 17

Caring for Feet

By Angela Evans
Consultant Podiatrist
Flinders Medical Centre and Ashford Medical Centre,
Adelaide

Many of the complications of diabetes may be due to lack of knowledge. Certainly, people with diabetes who develop problems with their feet are often unaware of how this is linked to their diabetes or of the many simple preventative measures which can be taken.

There are essentially two changes which can occur during diabetes which will directly affect foot health.

These are Nerve Damage *(Neuropathy)* and *Damage of Blood Vessels* in legs and feet *(Peripheral Vascular Disease)*. Both have been associated with persistently high blood glucose levels which means that you should aim at control of diabetes in order to avoid problems.

Medical evidence shows that long-term control of diabetes through regular exercise and low fat diet plus no-smoking and moderate alcohol intake reduces the severity of these conditions and may remove the risk totally.

Nerve and blood vessel damage affects foot health in a number of ways.

Nerve damage (neuropathy) can occur when diabetes is poorly controlled for a long time. This puts the feet at great risk of being damaged, because nerves are our emergency warning system.

Normal healthy feet have nerves which give good sensation to every part of the foot and leg. It is because of these nerves that we are able to feel things affecting the feet, such as tight shoes, sharp objects, hot water and an in-grown toenail or corn.

It is the pain or discomfort from such things which is transmitted by the nerves, alerting us to danger and protecting us from hurting ourselves.

If these nerves are not doing their job, we are not alerted to potential danger and the feet are at risk. Therefore it is most important to know how well the nerves are functioning and how much extra care must be taken. The podiatrist or doctor will carry out tests to ascertain the level of sensitivity.

Sometimes people with diabetes notice uncomfortable feelings in their legs and feet. These have been described as "pins and needles", a burning sensation or itchiness.

These often feel worse at night. People feeling such discomfort should contact their doctor, as a review of diabetic control may be necessary.

Many people report such sensations before they even know they have diabetes, and often the feelings will disappear when the diabetes is brought under control.

Apart from high blood glucose levels causing nerve damage, high alcohol consumption and a diet lacking in vitamin B may also aggravate nerve function.

As with nerve damage, Blood Vessel Damage or Peripheral Vascular Disease can be caused by blood glucose levels which are too high for too long but unlike nerve damage, which is specific to people with diabetes, damage to the blood vessels can affect anyone.

Also known as "clogging" or narrowing of the arteries, this condition means the amount of blood able to flow through the blood vessels is reduced. This occurs more quickly in the feet and legs where arteries are smaller, and the longer it continues, the further the arteries will narrow, meaning the feet will not receive enough blood to keep them healthy.

The factors which promote clogging include smoking, high fat diet, lack of exercise, high

Caring for Feet

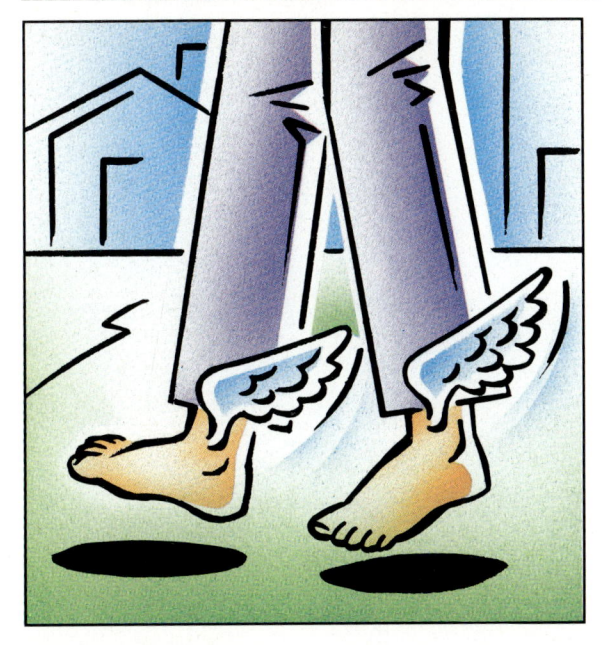

blood pressure and, in the case of people with diabetes, high blood glucose levels.

In such a case, where the feet are not healthy due to lack of blood supply, they are more prone to infection following any injury which breaks the skin.

Skin is a very important protective barrier between your feet and infections – more so under these conditions, and so dry skin which breaks more easily must be avoided through regular use of moisturising creams.

In trying to avoid infections of this nature, it must be remembered that the effects of infections can go far beyond the foot and in fact can actually cause high blood glucose levels. This in turn will lower resistance to infections. Therefore it is important to seek medical attention if blood glucose levels are high – especially if you have a foot injury and possible infection.

Just as important as knowing how good the sensation in your feet is, it is vital to know if you have enough blood circulating.

Signs of poor blood supply can include sharp cramps after walking short distances or up stairs, pain in the feet even at rest, feet feeling cold, feet looking a reddish-blue colour and cuts which are slow to heal.

Any of these symptoms should be checked by your podiatrist or doctor.

It is important to note however, that if you have nerve damage you will not be able to feel any of the signs which indicate poor circulation and it will need to be determined by the podiatrist or doctor.

Most of the causes of blood vessel damage can be reduced by your action, with the help of your dietitian and doctor. Taking affirmative action early may well avoid serious blood vessel damage – or stop it getting to a critical stage.

Footcare and footwear

Once you know how much sensation and blood supply your feet have, the issues of foot care and footwear become a lot clearer.

People with totally insensitive feet and a poor blood flow have to be extremely careful if they are to avoid limb threatening problems.

For these people, on a daily basis, the feet must be:
- well washed and dried gently.
- moisturised with a good cream.
- checked for trouble spots such as redness, swelling, cuts, pus discharge, splinters or blisters – being especially careful to look between toes, around the heels and nail edges and at the sole of the foot. If eyesight is poor, a family member or friend should check for you.
- covered in a clean sock or stocking preferably non-synthetic, which does not have rough seams.
- protected in a shoe which fits well and has been checked for stones, pins, buttons or anything else which could cause damage.

If you have good sensation in your feet and adequate blood circulation, good foot care is generally the same as recommended for everyone.
- Hygiene is always important. Make sure feet are dried well after a bath or shower, particularly between the toes where moisture can lead to tinea.
- If the skin is too dry, use a good moisturiser.
- Socks or stockings should be clean, with wool or cotton providing better ventilation.
- Shoes are worn to protect the feet. To do this

properly the shoe must be well-fitting. Shoes that are too big, too small, too tight or otherwise unsuitable for your feet can cause blisters, corns and nail problems. So make sure your shoe fits and is appropriate for the activity you are undertaking. Your podiatrist can advise you on the best shoe for your requirements.

It is often said a person with diabetes should never walk barefoot or cut their own toenails.

Certainly this is true for anyone who has lost sensation in their feet, as they could step on something sharp, cut their foot and not be aware of it. If this person also has reduced blood circulation, this could lead to infection and perhaps even turn gangrenous. In such a case a well-fitting shoe could have prevented a disaster.

Similarly, it is a risk for anyone with poor circulation or bad sensation to cut their own nails. Also, problem nails that are thickened or tend to be "in-grown" should be seen to by a podiatrist. Cut your own nails only if you can see well, reach your feet easily, and have good blood circulation.

Nails should be cut straight across, not too short and never down the sides. Rough edges can be filed with an emery board.

Other problems such as recurrent ankle sprains, corns and calluses, clawed toes and leg soreness should all be investigated by a podiatrist. Many of these problems are due to an unstable foot structure following a breakdown in the foot's mechanical framework.

Anything such as this can make exercising difficult and should be checked.

Things to avoid

"Corn-cure" chemicals are not only wrongly named, they are dangerous. Corns are due to excess pressure, so see a podiatrist to find out why this is happening and how it can be prevented. Strong corrosive acids such as are found in corn-cures have no place on anyone's feet and should never be used.

Radiators and hot water bottles can also be dangerous. Someone without sensation in their feet can receive serious burns without realising it. Keep a safe distance from radiators and use a knee rug if still cold.

Hot bitumen and sand in summer can seriously burn feet if sensation is lost.

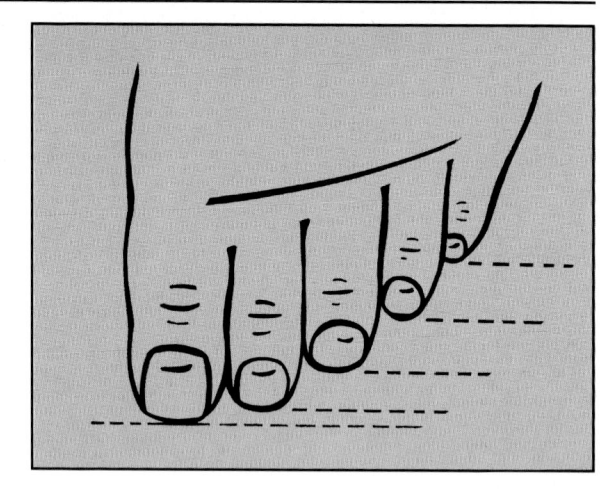

Nails should be cut straight across, not too short and never down the sides.

Foot First aid

If you have normal sensation in your feet, you will feel injuries if they occur but if not, you'll find them only when you inspect your feet each day.

On finding an injury:
• wash and dry the injured area
• apply a good antiseptic
• cover with a sterile dressing

It is important to always have dressings and antiseptic at hand. Your podiatrist, pharmacist, doctor or nurse will be able to advise on the best products.

If there is no improvement in 24 hours, seek professional help.

❑   ❑   ❑

While a broad rule can be applied to the types of problems and their treatment, the needs of every person with diabetes are individual and therefore it is essential to visit a podiatrist or doctor for complete assessment.

They will be able to advise specifically on the necessary foot care. This assessment should be done each year, or as directed.

Foot problems can be a side-effect of diabetes but with early assessment and proper care there is no reason why they cannot be overcome. It is very possible to have healthy feet with diabetes – it is up to you.

CHAPTER 18

Diabetes and Pregnancy

By Dr Ian Martin
Consultant Physician, Diabetes Clinic, Royal Womens Hospital
Endocrinologist, Royal Melbourne Hospital
and Dr Alison Nankervis
Physician, Diabetes Clinic, Royal Womens Hospital
Endocrinologist, Royal Melbourne Hospital

Recent advances in the treatment of diabetes have been such that pregnancy in women with diabetes usually results in a normal delivery with no effects on the mother's long term health.

The outlook for the baby is also excellent, but this depends on close co-operation between the woman and the medical team caring for her before and during pregnancy.

Some women are found to have diabetes during pregnancy without it ever having been suspected before. In these cases management is usually less demanding than for the woman with diabetes and the pregnancy should result in the delivery of a normal baby.

Metabolic changes dumg pregnancy

In order to better understand the care required, it is necessary to have a knowledge of the metabolic changes the woman with diabetes will undergo during pregnancy.

Early in pregnancy it is not uncommon for the mother's body to become more efficient in using glucose and thus for insulin requirements to drop slightly.

Then, by about the fifth or sixth month, the placenta – the baby's source of nutrition, has increased in size and begins to contribute significantly to the production of oestrogens and other hormones which antagonise the effect of insulin.

This means a state of temporary insulin resistance is produced in the latter half of pregnancy.

In addition, the demands of the growing baby are such that the mother is more prone to use ketones, the normal products of the liver which are part of the process of fatty acid breakdown, and fats. These changes mean that the woman requiring insulin may need higher doses or more frequent injections to enable the growing baby to obtain the nutrition and carbohydrate diet it requires.

The changes can also cause a deterioration in glucose tolerance in women who are susceptible to diabetes but have not actually suffered from it previously.

In these cases a temporary state of diabetes known as gestational diabetes can develop, most commonly after the 24th week of pregnancy.

After the baby is born and the placenta delivered, these changes are rapidly reversed so that insulin requirements fall dramatically and the temporary diabetes will usually end.

Pregnancy in women with pre-existing diabetes

These women usually have Type 1 diabetes although some – particularly over the age of 30, may have Type 2 diabetes, managed by diet, exercise and tablets.

Women with Type 2 diabetes can be reassured by the fact that while it is not usual to use oral tablets during pregnancy, there is no evidence that they are harmful to the development of the foetus. As the chapter *Use of Tablets* points out, insulin is the preferred treatment for pregnant women with pre-existing Type 2 diabetes.

It is important that early medical consultation is sought once pregnancy is confirmed. The medical team is often a physician and obstetrician with special interest in diabetes, a neonatal paediatrician and where possible, a dietitian and diabetes nurse.

While it is not always possible to have this whole team, the women with known diabetes will require specialist care and advice.

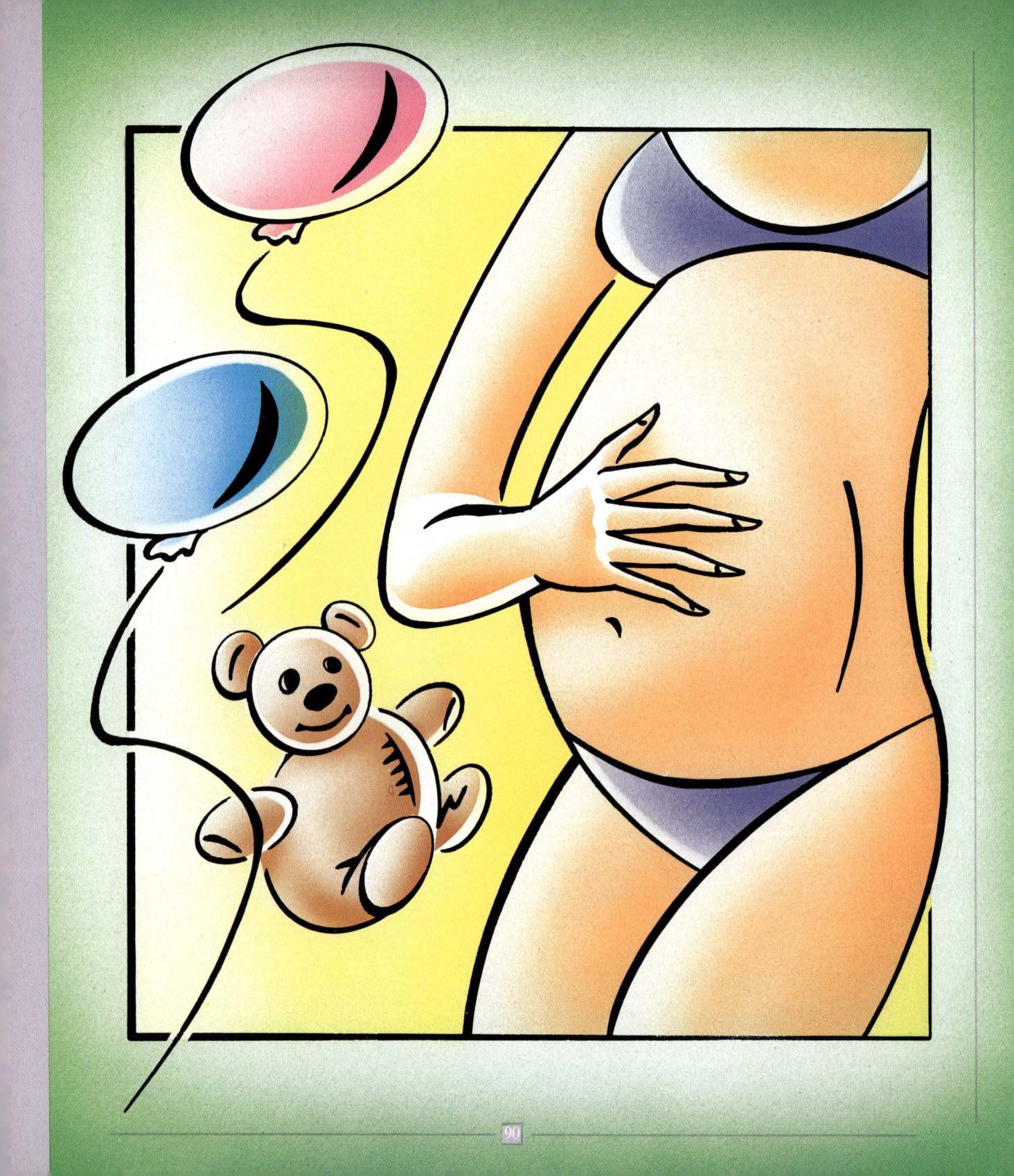

Diabetes and Pregnancy

Throughout the pregnancy, the aim is to achieve excellent control of diabetes. Control of diabetes at the time of conception is important, but the particular insulin schedule used may require modification during pregnancy.

There is no absolute rule for the type of insulin treatment during pregnancy. Individual assessment is necessary but it is usual for twice daily or more frequent insulin injections to be used from early pregnancy.

Later in pregnancy when insulin requirements rise, further modification may be necessary, depending on the degree of control the woman has achieved. This should be discussed with the physician.

It is important the diet is not restricted unduly and that carbohydrate content in particular is adequate.

An overly restricted carbohydrate intake can accentuate ketosis – where too many ketones are produced and passed in the urine. This, if severe, can be harmful in pregnancy.

In early pregnancy, morning sickness and loss of appetite may present practical difficulties which can usually be helped by smaller, more frequent meals. In late pregnancy further modifications to diet may be required and throughout pregnancy the advice of a dietitian is helpful in ensuring diet is adequate for both mother and baby.

Urine tests in pregnancy often show glucose at lower than usual blood glucose levels and so are of little value except to monitor the presence of ketones.

The more accepted method of monitoring control of diabetes is blood glucose testing. Ideally levels between 3 and 8 mmol/l should be achieved between meals but individual levels may vary.

The glycated haemoglobin (Hb AlC) or fructosamine value estimates average blood glucose and is very useful in assessing overall diabetic control, so it may be done more frequently during pregnancy.

All these matters should be discussed with the physician at an early stage of pregnancy.

As well as regular checks of weight and blood pressure, women with diabetes will require regular eye tests for retinopathy and of the kidneys for proteinuria and function.

The obstetrician will usually arrange an ultrasound examination of the baby within the first four months of pregnancy and then as required, to estimate the baby's physical growth and development.

Towards the end of pregnancy other means of monitoring the baby's health, such as examination of the heart beat by a cardiotachograph, oestrogen estimations in blood or urine and amniocentesis may be carried out.

These days it is not usually necessary to admit the pregnant woman with diabetes to hospital for any prolonged period. However, admissions may be necessary early in pregnancy for re-stabilisation, at any time if there is an acute infection or other illness with diabetic control, and in late pregnancy before delivery.

High blood pressure or excess fluid may also require hospitalisation.

Women with pre-existing diabetes on diet with or without tablets, will often require insulin during pregnancy.

In these cases it is usual for diabetic control and diet to be assessed early in pregnancy and then monitored throughout. When the increased insulin requirements of mid-pregnancy occur the previous control may become inadequate and insulin will be needed for the second half of pregnancy.

The management will be similar to that of the woman with Type 1 diabetes and following delivery control of diabetes may be possible by diet alone.

Common concerns about pregnancy and the baby

All women are naturally concerned that their baby will be healthy and normal. Very often this anxiety is greater in women with diabetes and certainly, in the past, women with diabetes had a poorer outcome of pregnancy.

It is true that women with diabetes still have a higher than normal risk of both malformation or miscarriage but this risk has decreased enormously and continues to improve. The chances of the baby born to a woman with diabetes being normal are excellent but it is now believed that good control of diabetes at the time of conception and early pregnancy is an important factor in reducing the overall risks.

Following birth – particularly if the baby is premature, it is usual for it to be monitored closely in a special nursery to avoid possible problems such as hypoglycaemia, jaundice or breathing difficulties.

Very often women are concerned that their babies will have diabetes. There is very little chance that this will occur in early life. The chances of this happening are discussed in full in Chapter 29, The Genetics of Diabetes.

The emphasis on control of diabetes during pregnancy does make the possibility of hypoglycaemia more likely. Fortunately low blood glucose levels do not appear to affect the baby, but severe hypoglycaemia of course should be avoided.

Very often women seem to adapt to low blood glucose levels in pregnancy so that adjustments to both the insulin schedule and diet will usually make it possible to have excellent control, particularly with the added motivation of maintaining good control during pregnancy.

Unexpected illness can cause loss of control and dehydration more quickly in pregnancy, so the woman must contact her physician immediately if she becomes ill.

For many years it has been usual to deliver the woman with Type 1 diabetes at 37-38 weeks gestation – about two weeks before term.

Attitudes in some centres have changed on this but practical experience, the individual assessment of the mother and the baby's health will determine each individual case.

Delivery may be normal vaginal – often following induction of labour, or by Caesarean section, depending on obstetric and individual indications.

The management of diabetes for either form of delivery is not a problem, and can be adapted as required with a combination of insulin and, if necessary, intravenous glucose to maintain carbohydrate intake.

Delivery must always be in a hospital with full facilities for the care of mother and baby.

Following delivery of baby and placenta, there is a dramatic fall in insulin requirements, which may last two or three days. The diabetes will then usually readjust and insulin requirements will return to near the prepregnancy level.

There is no medical reason why women with diabetes should not breast feed. If they had been taking oral hypoglycaemic tablets before pregnancy, they can stay on insulin treatment while breast feeding.

Presence of complications in the mother

As explained in Chapter 16, eye disease is a common side effect of diabetes and is not generally of great concern during pregnancy. Most authorities believe there is no significant deterioration in retinopathy during pregnancy, but eyes should always be examined regularly.

If necessary, laser treatment can be carried out during pregnancy without any ill effects.

Kidney disease is of more concern and requires individual assessment.

Pre-eclampsia – the development of high blood pressure, swelling and eventually protein in the urine, can be a problem in any pregnancy. It can also occur in women with diabetes particularly Type 1 diabetes, and may require earlier hospitalisation and delivery than expected.

The obstetrician and physician will advise if there are any problems in this regard.

Urinary infections are also potentially serious in pregnancy and any symptoms or unexplained fevers should be reported early.

Planned pregnancy

For all the reasons already stated, it is important that the woman with diabetes plans her pregnancy and has her diabetes under control when she conceives.

Prior discussion with the physician is a good idea and some special clinics for pre-pregnancy counselling are available.

If oral contraception is being used, it is best to make plans before the Pill is ceased.

Diabetes developing during pregnancy

At least three women in every hundred and in some racial groups such as Aborigines and

Diabetes and Pregnancy

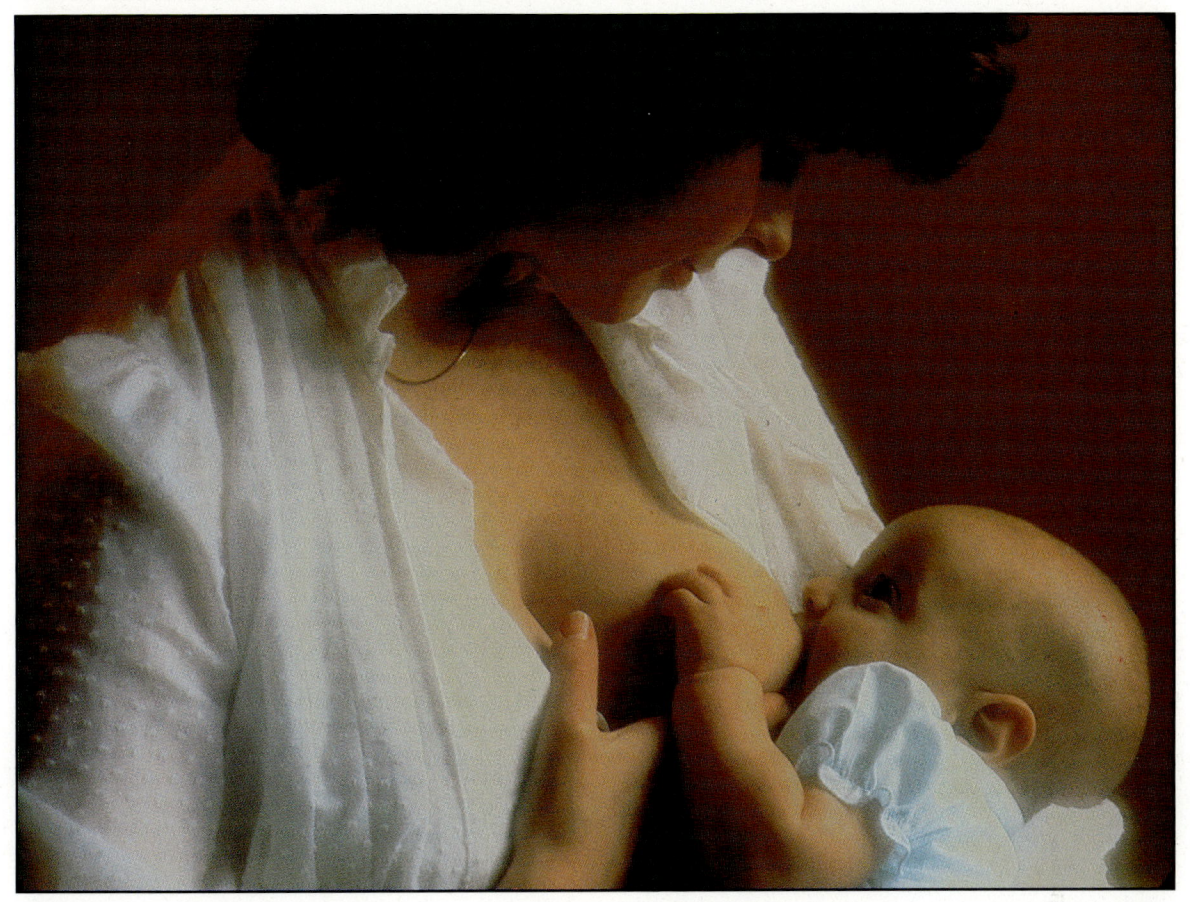

Vietnamese even more, will develop diabetes during pregnancy, .

This form of diabetes is known as Gestational Diabetes and, as discussed, usually develops in the latter half of pregnancy and will improve after delivery.

Some women may be found to have previously unrecognised diabetes when undergoing routine tests in early pregnancy.

Gestational diabetes is more common in women aged over 30, particularly when there is a family history of Type 2 diabetes and overweight.

It is usually recognised during routine testing of urine, but testing blood glucose to detect gestational diabetes is currently being recommended as cases of gestational diabetes may be missed by routine urine testing or only detected towards the end of pregnancy.

Diabetes in pregnancy is confirmed by a glucose tolerance test, exactly the same as for non-pregnant people.

The treatment of the condition depends upon the severity of the abnormality of glucose metabolism. In many women this is relatively mild and treatment by diet alone is sufficient.

The diet will restrict total calories but ensure adequate carbohydrate intake is preserved. It will also be aimed at controlling the woman's weight.

Too strict a diet can impair nutrition and promote excess ketosis, so the advice of a dietitian is very helpful.

If the condition is more severe and blood glucose cannot be controlled by diet, insulin will be required for the duration of pregnancy. This will be commenced under instructions of the medical team and in most cases other tests such

Diabetes and Pregnancy

as glycated haemoglobin, kidney function and blood pressure will be carried out as a matter of routine. Provided there is no other reason why it should not, the pregnancy will be over a normal 38-40 week gestational period and delivery by normal means. The condition of gestational diabetes often remits following delivery but will persist in some women who will then require continuing treatment.

In those women whose diabetes goes away after delivery, a follow up glucose tolerance test will be carried out six to eight weeks after delivery.

Even if this test proves normal, these women have a much higher than normal chance of developing diabetes in later life. For this reason a sensible diet and regular exercise to avoid overweight are important.

These women should inform their general practitioner that they may be at risk of developing diabetes in later life.

The woman with diabetes should approach pregnancy with high expectations. Successful outcome depends on close co-operation with the medical team and will require more frequent than usual visits and checks.

❏ ❏ ❏

As with any pregnant woman, it is important she ask questions about her worries and concerns and seeks advice in the event of any sudden infection or deterioration of diabetic control.

If this is done, and the woman takes a sensible and disciplined approach to her pregnancy, there is no reason it should not be an enjoyable and rewarding experience, with a beautiful baby to show for it.

CHAPTER 19

Diabetes and Female Sexuality

By Dr Lesley Campbell
Deputy Director
St Vincents Diabetes Centre
Sydney

Despite being a topic of great importance, the effects of diabetes upon female sexuality is an area about which not enough is known. In fact, there is much more information about the potential sexual problems of men than women with diabetes.

This is of course not an easy topic for accurate research. People are often shy about discussing intimate matters with others and there are no simple tests of sexual function in women. However, the major part of the limited evidence indicates that there is no reason why women with diabetes should have more sexual difficulties than other women.

Regardless of whether a woman has diabetes or not, there are a multitude of factors both physical and emotional which contribute to a satisfactory sexual life.

Any woman can have difficulties in any step in the sequence of sexual desire, sexual arousal and orgasm. This may be one reason that about two out of four normal women with otherwise happy and satisfying marriages will, if asked, report the presence of a sexual problem.

Emotional factors (like depression and marital conflict) and physical factors (like menopause or chronic illness) can all cause some type of sexual dysfunction.

On the emotional side, some studies do suggest that diabetes developing in later life can have a detrimental effect on the whole marital relationship, including sexual desire and satisfaction. The woman with late onset diabetes may be at a vulnerable time in her life and may feel less attractive, less healthy and subsequently be less sexually responsive. On the other hand, in couples where diabetes was present before the relationship, the partnership may be stronger because the man has knowingly accepted the implications of his partner's diabetes.

As far as the physical effects of diabetes are concerned, high blood glucose levels can have a temporary adverse effect on many aspects of a woman's life: she may feel tired, less interested in sexual activity and less able to enjoy it. These symptoms will respond to a sustained improvement in blood glucose levels and therefore it is worthwhile to assess the effect of improved blood glucose control on such symptoms.

While some men with diabetes who have secondary damage to the nerves or circulation are known to develop impotence, there is no corresponding sexual difficulty found in women with such complications. There may be some lessening of vaginal lubrication in such cases, but that problem is easily treated by use of a lubricant. Even when women with advanced nerve damage are compared to other women without such damage, there is usually no difference in sexual function.

While it seems that diabetes does not generally cause extra sexual problems in women, when asked many women will report some sexual problem. Usually such problems can be helped by suitable sexual counselling - that is, private discussion and advice over several sessions with a trained counsellor.

❏ ❏ ❏

Any woman who is worried about some aspect of her sexual relationship should seek help. Her local doctor or diabetes specialist will be aware of a suitable counsellor for confidential treatment.

A happy sexual life is one of the most pleasant aspects of a successful relationship. Generally women with diabetes can enjoy a healthy and satisfying sex life.

CHAPTER 20

Sexual Problems in Men

By Dr Ted Keogh
Medical Director,
Reproductive Medicine Research Institute
Queen Elizabeth II Medical Centre
Perth

There are two main sexual problems which affect men with diabetes — Impotence and Retrograde Ejaculation.

Impotence is when the man is unable to achieve an erection adequate for intercourse – a condition which makes the man despair, frustrates and angers his partner, often leading to an uncomfortable home environment for the children.

Retrograde Ejaculation is a condition in which semen flows the wrong way, ending up in the bladder, which, while not affecting normal sexual relations, can make it difficult to produce a child.

Impotence

The penis contains two rods of spongy tissue lying side by side. On the undersurface is a tube – the urethra, which conveys urine from the bladder. The rods of tissue can become filled with blood, converting the soft flaccid penis to a hard, rod-like appendage.

This "erection" occurs when the valves in the arteries delivering blood to the spongy tissue in the shaft of the penis open up, filling the many tiny cavities which make up the tissue.

These events are under nervous control. When a man contemplates sexual activity, messages travel from the brain down the spinal cord and through nerves to open the "valves".

If a man becomes anxious while he has an erection, the valves may close. Thus a psychologically stressed patient, irrespective of the presence of diabetes, can't achieve an erection.

The onset of impotence can be a gradual process starting with the softening of erections, then a tendency to ejaculate prematurely, inability to sustain erections and finally the inability to initiate an erection.

The process may be protracted, over a decade or occur relatively rapidly over 12 months. If the situation of the relationship is tense it is more likely to develop sooner.

Such a condition is often one of the early metabolic side effects of diabetes and therefore it will not be accompanied by other abnormal features which point to diabetes – such as neuropathy, peripheral vascular disease and skin lesions of the feet.

The main test is a diagnostic intracavernosal injection of medication. The copora cavernosa is the spongy tissue which engorges with blood. When medications which open up the blood vessels – or vasodilators, are injected into this space the arteries leading into the cavities fill them with blood.

About 5-10 minutes after injection the penis becomes erect for half an hour or so.

If this injection test fails, the cause is probably a blockage of the arteries supplying the penis.

X-rays can also be used, with dye injected into arteries leading to the penis. Occasionally blockages are operated upon in the same way obstructed arteries are bypassed in heart surgery.

Treatment

The most common first line of treatment in Australia is an explanation of the cause of failure and, where possible, reassurance that the problem is not psychological.

It is not possible at the outset to be confident about what proportion of the cause is physical and what proportion is psychological.

Sexual Problems in Men

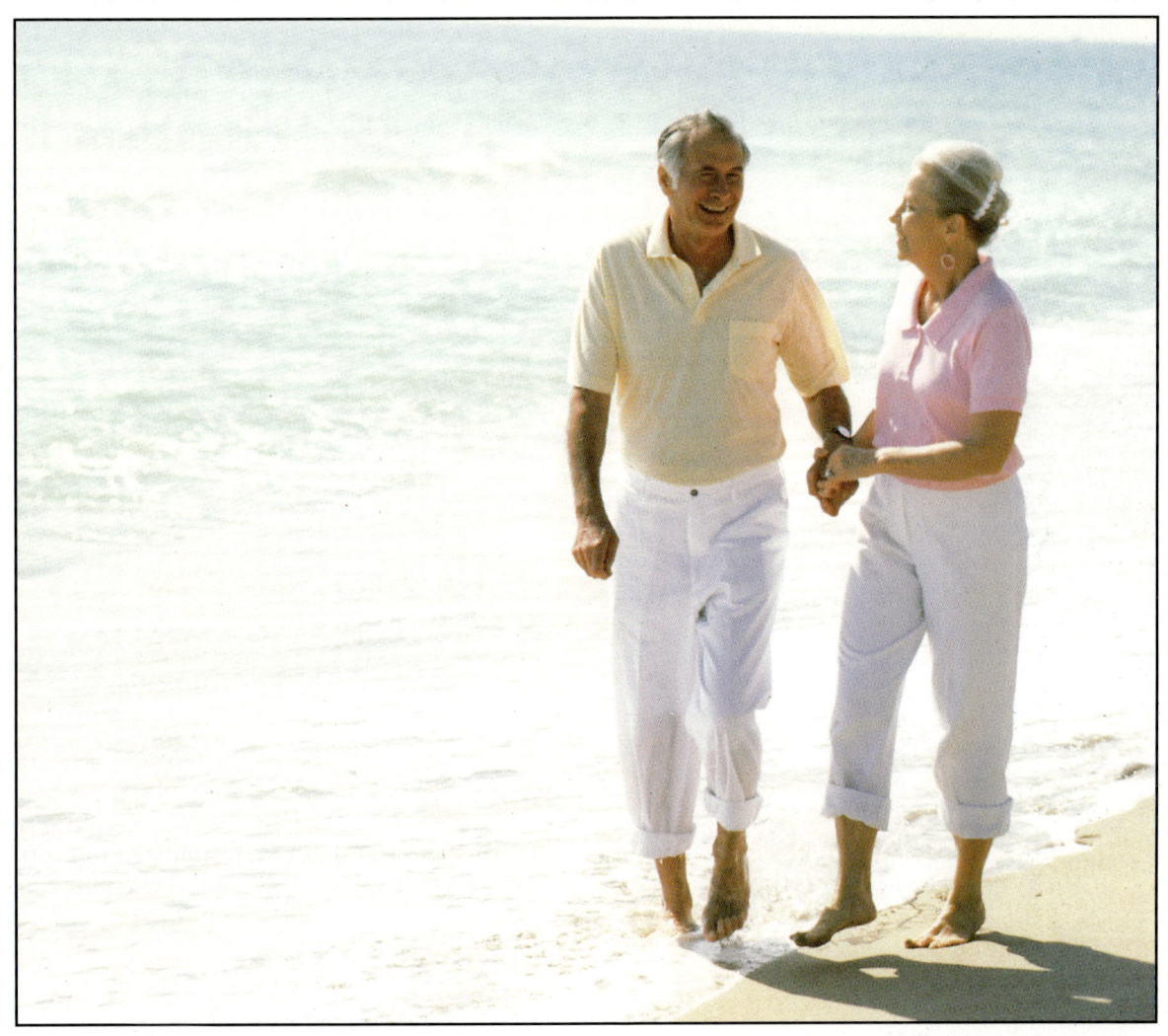

Until the mid 1970's, many doctors believed impotence was 95 per cent psychological and because of this many men still hold this view. However, as more precise means of diagnosis have become available, this ratio has decreased and is now believed to be 50-50.

When some men commence insulin treatment they observe a striking improvement in their erections.

This implies that restoration of normal glucose metabolism has a beneficial effect on either the nerves, smooth muscle or blood vessels, permitting normal intercourse. However at a later stage some men find their capacity to have intercourse is severely compromised or nonexistent.

Penile injection

The impotent patient is usually invited to try the injection technique as a way of creating an erection – and although often initially unwilling, patients are surprised to find the treatment almost painless.

Penile implant

For some people the fuss over the injection detracts from the spontaneity of love making and for this reason they request a penile implant.

Sexual Problems in Men

Implants are available in two types, the first being malleable rods of a metal core surrounded by an inert rubber such as silicone. The penis can be bent down, or straightened for intercourse, although a disadvantage is a bulge in front of the trousers because the penis is permanently rigid and partly erect.

Another type of implant is an inflatable device consisting of two sausage shaped balloons in the shaft of the penis, one in each spongy cavity. A reservoir of water is placed in front of the bladder and a pump located in the scrotum. The pump can be manually worked, filling the balloons with water, and causing an erection.

After recovery from surgery, it is almost impossible to distinguish the penis from normal in either the flaccid or erect state. Disadvantages are the costs, at around $5000, complex surgery and the potential for mechanical failure.

Although no synthetic device can ever replace nature, satisfaction with both kinds of implant has been excellent.

Vacuum Device

Vacuum erection devices have been available in one form or another for more than a century. The current versions consist of a perspex cylinder which fits over the penis and rests on the skin of the pubic area. A hand pump-generated vacuum is created around the penis which draws blood into the shaft of the penis.

After applying an elastic band to the base to trap the blood the perspex cylinder is removed leaving the penis engorged.

Retrograde ejaculation

The other common condition is Retrograde Ejaculation – failure of contraction of the bladder neck sphincter and forward propulsion of semen through the urethral opening. The semen flows the wrong way, ending up in the bladder.

The first symptom of this condition is a reduced volume of semen, or none, despite normal sensations of orgasm. When the man passes urine after orgasm he may notice a cloudy discolouration and sperm are evident under a microscope.

When infertility is treated ejaculation is timed to coincide with ovulation, determined by temperature charts and hormone levels in the woman's blood. Viable sperm may be retreived from the bladder by voiding after ejaculation.

Other options include medications such as ephedrine and brompheniramine.

The disorder is common among men who have had prostate surgery, and does not interfere with their sexual function.

❏ ❏ ❏

In summary, diabetes does cause sexual problems in men, but modern treatment has a lot to offer.

CHAPTER 21

You and Your Health Care Team

By Dr Pat Phillips,
Director, Endocrine and Diabetes Service
The Queen Elizabeth Hospital, Adelaide
and Dr June Raine, Assistant State Director
Royal Australian College of General Practitioners, Family Medicine Program
New South Wales

The team approach

You are living with diabetes 24 hours a day, 365 days a year with no holidays. You are balancing food, exercise and medication and trying to keep in control. Fortunately, you don't have to face it alone.

In Australia there are a range of health care professionals to help you handle your diabetes. Your health professionals usually work as a team, each bringing special skills and knowledge to your total health care plan.

The most important member and the leader of the team, is **you**. It is easy for your doctor, diabetes nurse or dietitian to lose track. You are often the only one who knows the whole picture – what has been done, what the problems are, what needs doing.

This chapter gives you some tips on how to lead the "Team Approach" to diabetes care (Diagram).

Your responsibilities

DAY-TO-DAY CARE:

Diet — You can become your own dietitian and use the available resources to develop a wide range of recipes. You can choose from a wide variety of foods.

Every now and then (eg; each birthday) – think about your food selection. If you feel limited or are limited in your food choices, consult your books and pamphlets and consider seeing your dietitian.

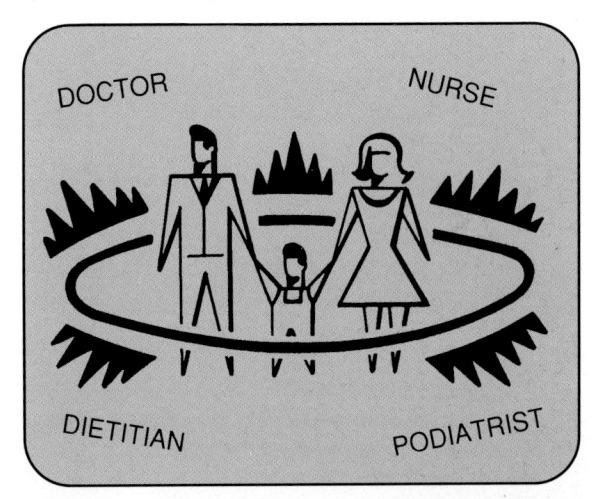

Weight — You are your own harshest critic. If you think you look OK in the mirror, your weight is probably fine. Weight records enable you to keep track of things and give you a warning that your weight is creeping up.

Exercise — A regular routine exercise programme is a good idea. In that way, you are likely to keep going and not let yourself slip back. If you exercise with a group (eg, through your local council), a friend, a family member or a dog, so much the better.

Medication — It's easy to run out, but you really shouldn't. Get a spare bottle and also keep your eye on the expiry dates. If you are on insulin, you may need some glucagon and someone in the house needs to be able to use it in an emergency.

You and Your Health Care Team

YEAR-TO-YEAR CARE:
Have you fully considered:
- Getting a medical alert bracelet, necklace, or card – so people can do the right thing even if you can't tell them.
- Joining the Ambulance Fund – so you won't get an enormous bill!
- Joining Diabetes Australia – so you can keep yourself up to date with new developments and learn of meetings, support groups, political efforts, education materials, etc.

Have you:
- Joined the National Diabetes Supplies Scheme which provides subsidised syringes and monitoring strips.
- Told the motor vehicles department and your insurance company that you have diabetes – thus avoiding breaking the law, or missing out on getting accident compensation.
- Had your tetanus toxoid status updated – you need an injection against tetanus each 10 years. (For example; each time you notch up a decade – age 20, 30, ... 100, 110 ....!).
- Had a vaccination against 'flu' or pneumonia. Perhaps you should ask your doctor if you need one.
- Arranged for follow-up by an ophthalmologist (at the intervals recommended).

You need to keep track of these things. Perhaps you could check through your responsibilities at least each year to make sure you are still ahead (perhaps on birthdays, Christmas or New Year).

Your doctor's responsibilities

Your doctor shares your aims – to keep you healthy. You should discuss your regular follow-up and arrange a schedule to suit you both. Some areas your doctor will be considering include:

1. **Diabetic Control – Glycated Haemoglobin/Fructosamine**

    You are responsible for managing and keeping track of the day-to-day control of your blood glucose level. Your doctor can check your long-term diabetic control by checking your haemoglobin A1c or glycated haemoglobin.

    Glucose in the blood attaches to blood proteins. The protein that carries oxygen is called haemoglobin and has a life of about 120 days. Normally about 6 per cent of haemoglobin has glucose attached to it and 94 per cent is free of glucose. The part with glucose attached is said to be "glycated" (glycos = glucose). If blood glucose levels are often high then more glucose attaches to haemoglobin (eg 15 per cent glycated).

    Since haemoglobin stays in the body for some time, this measurement reflects all the "Highs" and "Lows" of blood glucose levels over the past weeks to months. The higher the average blood glucose, the higher the glycated haemoglobin. One reading gives an average blood glucose over the long-term. The test can be done by your general practitioner every 3-4 months to check your overall control.

    Similarly fructosamine measurements assess glucose attached to other blood proteins and reflects diabetes control over the preceding few weeks.

2. **Blood Pressure**

    People with diabetes often have high blood pressure which puts an extra strain on blood vessels. Imagine the effects of pounding the delicate tissues 100,000 times per day. That's the number of times your heart beats each day.

    As the heart contracts and pumps blood out, the pressure in the blood vessels rises to a peak (systolic blood pressure). The empty heart then fills up with blood and the pressure falls to a trough (diastolic blood pressure). In general the lower the blood pressure the better. Your aim is to get values under 140 systolic and 90 diastolic. (Blood pressure is recorded like this: 140/90).

    Once again your doctor will want to check your blood pressure at regular intervals.

3. **Eyes (see Chapter 16)**

    Visual Acuity
    This can be checked each year when you get

You and Your Health Care Team

DATE	FEB	JUNE	OCT	FEB	JUNE	OCT	FEB	JUNE	OCT
GENERAL Weight									
BP									
Glycated haemoglobin									
EYES Visual acuity									
Ophthalmologist due in									
KIDNEYS Microalbuminuria									
Dipstick									
Creatinine									
FEET Arteries									
Nerves									
INJECTION SITE									
VACCINATIONS									
Due in									

your licence renewal. Visual acuity is recorded as a fraction. 6/6 means that when you are six meters away you can read the chart designed to be read at six meters. 6/9 or 6/12 would mean that at six meters away you can't read the six meter chart and can only read the one designed to be read at nine or 12 meters away. You should keep your own record of your visual acuity.

Ophthalmologist
Diabetes Australia recommends that your doctor refer you to an ophthalmologist for review. Only an ophthalmologist can fully test your eyes. After the initial assessment, follow-up can be at intervals suggested by the ophthalmologist.

We recommend initial assessment for people with diabetes
- More than 30 years – at the time diabetes is diagnosed
- Less than 30 years – 5 years after the diagnosis of diabetes.

4. **Kidneys (see Chapter 15)**

A check of the protein in your urine will give an early indication of diabetic kidney problems.

The first sign of kidney damage is often the

appearance of a very small amount of protein (albumin) in the urine. This <u>small</u> (micro) amount of <u>albumin</u> in <u>urine</u> is called <u>microalbuminuria</u> and can be detected by special tests. At this stage, damage is reversible.

A check with a special test strip will warn of silent urinary tract infection.

Your doctor might perform a blood test to check the level of waste products (creatinine or urea levels).

5. **Feet (see Chapter 17)**

   If you are not able to care for your feet, you should see a podiatrist regularly. Your doctor is interested in checking to make sure your pulses are still as good as ever (this means that the blood circulation is OK). He might also check that your sensation is still satisfactory so that, when you are damaging your feet, you can feel it and then stop doing the damage. A yearly check is wise.

6. **Injection Site (if you are on Insulin)**

   You are responsible for giving the injections properly (preferably in the abdominal wall) and for making sure you rotate the injection site so that you don't keep hitting the same spots. Your doctor is interested to make sure you are not getting any lumps or hollows which could affect the absorption of the insulin. A regular yearly check is enough.

Keeping track of your care

You may be seeing your doctor several times a year and it's easy for him and you to lose track of what has and has not been done. Many people find a log book a useful place to record the monitoring procedures.

A final word

Remember, <u>YOU</u> are the most important member of your health care team. You lead the "Team Approach" to diabetes care.

You and Your Health Care Team

Health Care Professionals

You may see various health professionals for help with specific problems. Sometimes it is confusing to keep the titles of the various specialists straight. This section is a glossary of health care professionals with whom you may come in contact. If you feel that you would like an appointment with one of these professionals, your doctor or another health care team member can refer you.

Dentist People with diabetes are at higher risk for periodontitis, a form of gum disease. It's good to make your dentist a member of your health care team. Have regular dental check-ups, and always tell any dentist you see that you have diabetes. Keep smiling!

Diabetes Nurse There are various kinds of nurses. Diabetes nurses provide in-patient and out-patient care and assessment, and will help you learn the knowledge and skills to control your diabetes.

Dietitian Provides dietary education, assessment and counselling regarding meal planning. Your dietitian will help you determine your nutritional requirements according to your weight, life-style, activity level, medication, and other health concerns. He or she can then help translate those requirements into specific meal plans for weight loss, fat and cholesterol and salt control.

Endocrinologist Medical specialist (physician) who treats people who have disorders of the endocrine glands, such as the pancreas. A "diabetologist" is another name for this team member.

General Practitioner A key member in the team. Your general practitioner will work with you and the other members to coordinate your care and ensure a consistent approach over the years ahead.

Obstetritian A specialist who cares for pregnant women. Some obstetritians have a special interest in diabetes during pregnancy.

Ophthalmologist Medical specialist who treats the eye. Your eye doctor will monitor any changes in your eyes, particularly those associated with diabetes, determine what those changes mean, and arrange any necessary treatment.

Optometrist Measures errors in refraction and prescribes glasses to correct the refractive errors.

Orthopaedic Surgeon A surgical specialist who treats the musculoskeletal system.

Paediatrician Medical specialist who treats children for various health problems.

Pharmacist A person licenced to prepare and dispense drugs and medicine. Your pharmacist knows of medications used in diabetic management and is a resource person for information about diabetes-care products.

Physical Therapist Uses physical measures (heat, cold, water, etc) to evaluate and treat disease and disability. Therapeutic exercises and training procedures are also used.

Podiatrist A professional trained in the treatment and prevention of foot disorders. Your podiatrist can advise and help you keep your feet healthy.

Psychiatrist Medical specialist who treats people who have emotional or psychological difficulties.

Psychologist Counsels people regarding psychological or emotional difficulties, also trained to conduct psychological testing.

Social Worker Counsels individuals and families regarding personal, family, or marital problems. Medical social workers also counsel people regarding the emotional aspects of illness. Social workers provide information as to community resources.

Urologist A surgical specialist in disorders of the urinary system, who can also help men who suffer with impotence.

Vascular Surgeon Surgical specialist who treats the blood vessels supplying body tissues.

DIABETES & YOU
An owner's manual

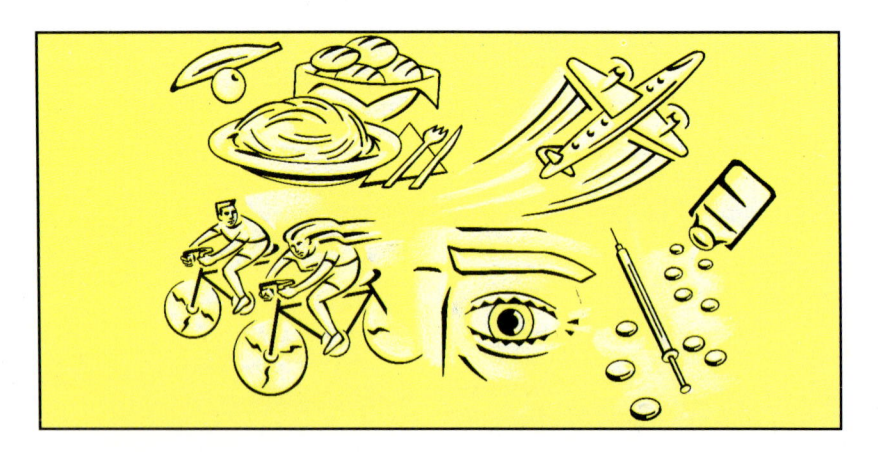

SPECIAL GROUPS

❏ The Schoolchild with Diabetes

Physical problems
Hypoglycaemia
Ketoacidosis
Food and Diabetes
Psychological problems
Children's Camps

❏ Diabetes – A Problem in Any Language

People
Material resources
Existing facilities

❏ Diabetes in Aborigines

Why are Aborigines so vulnerable to diabetes
Reversing the process
Implications for white people with Type 2 Diabetes

CHAPTER 22

The Schoolchild with Diabetes

By Prof Martin Silink
Director, Ray Williams Institute of
Paediatric Endocrinology, Diabetes & Metabolism
The Children's Hospital
Sydney

The formative early years at school are difficult enough for a child under normal circumstances, let alone with the added burden of diabetes.

The quality of the school experience is very important for all children. It helps them develop self-esteem and the ability to inter-relate with others, as well as equipping them with knowledge and problem solving abilities.

For this reason the vital role of the teacher and parent at this important time can never be under-estimated.

This is not to say that the teacher should consider the child with diabetes as a "problem child" or "poor learner". Diabetes does not decrease a child's ability to succeed academically, and in some case it can have the opposite effect.

The same standards of behaviour in the classroom should be expected from a child with diabetes as from any other child.

As with all kids, children with diabetes need to be accepted by their peer group and hate to be considered "different." For this reason, children with diabetes should be encouraged to participate in all school activities, including sport.

This said, it is true that having a child with diabetes in a class will mean added responsibility for the teacher.

The first step to coping with this responsibility is to have a basic understanding of diabetes. A description of the disorder and its treatment can be found in the early chapters of this book.

These chapters will give a basic grounding but to adequately cope with a child with diabetes, further action is recommended. While teachers do not receive any specific training on how to cope with what is often termed a "diabetic emergency", many of the larger childrens' hospitals can arrange for an expert to lecture teachers and ancillary staff.

Parents should also attend such lectures.

Sessions such as these are to be encouraged because it is important that the teacher be aware of the two types of problems – physical and psychological, that the child with diabetes faces.

While it is important that the child is generally not treated differently from other children, it is equally important that the teacher know the warning signs and what steps to take in an urgent situation.

Physical problems

Physically, there are four main areas in which special allowances must be made for children with diabetes.
- They may need to drink and urinate more often than others, as excessive thirst and urination are often the first clues to the diagnosis of diabetes and may recur whenever the blood sugar level rises for more than a few hours.
- They may need to be allowed to eat – either food, sugar or even sweets, at times different to others, even in class or at assembly. Of course requirements should be checked with the parent or doctor.
- Occasionally they may need to measure their blood glucose levels or take additional doses of insulin at school.
- They need to be checked for signs of hypoglycaemia or insulin reaction which, if untreated, may lead to unconsciousness.

Hypoglycaemia – the warning signs

Most people with diabetes experience a

"hypo" now and then and suffer no long term ill effects.

In children the blood sugar level is generally more erratic than in adults. A child may have a different reaction on different occasions but if there is an inexplicable change in colour, mood, attention or manner in a child with diabetes, suspect hypoglycaemia.

It is important that the teacher be aware that the child having a hypo is not responsible for his or her actions.

The symptoms to watch out for are:
- Headaches. There are no special features of these headaches but, as most children get headaches very infrequently, do not dismiss the symptom lightly. Parents should be aware that a child waking at night with a headache may be about to suffer a mild hypo or has had a low blood sugar while asleep.
- Changes in mood. These may range from outbursts of anger to a tendency to cry or unreasonable irritability. Once again remember, if caused by a hypo these are beyond the child's control.
- Lack of attention. A child suffering a hypo may appear well but seem to be daydreaming. The difference is that children suffering a hypo cannot be snapped out of their trance easily.
- Lack of energy or feeling of shakiness. These symptoms come on suddenly – over 5-10 minutes.
- Nausea and pains in the stomach. The pains may be constant or cramping. The feeling of nausea will make the child unwilling to eat but sugar must be given.
- Sudden pallor, with or without perspiration. The perspiration is usually visible but fairly subtle, causing the skin to feel clammy. It affects the whole body, not just the face.
- Drowsiness, listlessness, lack of concentration, change of consciousness. This may progress to complete unconsciousness and even to fitting if allowed to go untreated.

Treatment of hypoglycaemia

The two most important facts about "hypos" are that they are usually preventable, and that they must be treated quickly.

At the first signs of any of the warning symptoms, the child must be given sugar.

All children with diabetes should carry food to treat hypos, such as jelly beans or glucose tablets, and it is a good idea for teachers to keep sweets handy for emergencies.

People with diabetes have been taught to be self-reliant and can feel the symptoms of a hypo coming on and know the best action to take. With young children however the symptoms can often come on very quickly, giving them little time to react.

In such a case it is up to the teacher to act quickly and, unless specifically told otherwise by the child's parent, the child should be given something sweet, like five or six jellybeans, two heaped teaspoons of sugar in a little water or half a glass of lemonade. This should be followed with some solid food such as a sandwich, biscuit or piece of fruit.

Within 15 minutes the child should have responded and be able to go on with usual activities.

It is important that a child should not be left alone after suffering a hypo. If the hypo has passed, the child should rejoin the class with as little fuss as possible and the parents subsequently notified.

The teacher should make a note for parents of the time of the hypo, the severity and the treatment, to enable a judgement to be made on whether the insulin dose needs adjusting.

If the child is still unwell after 15 minutes, another dose of sugar followed by solid food should be given. If there is still no improvement, the parents or a doctor should be called.

The child should never be sent home alone after an attack but must always be collected by parents.

Treating severe hypoglycaemia

If the hypo progresses rapidly, or if the early warning signs were not detected, the child may become very drowsy, falling almost into a stupor, or even have a convulsion.

If the child can swallow, he or she should be encouraged to take sugar in an easily absorbed form, such as two to four heaped teaspoons of sugar in water, or a glass of lemonade.

As soon as the child is able to eat he/she

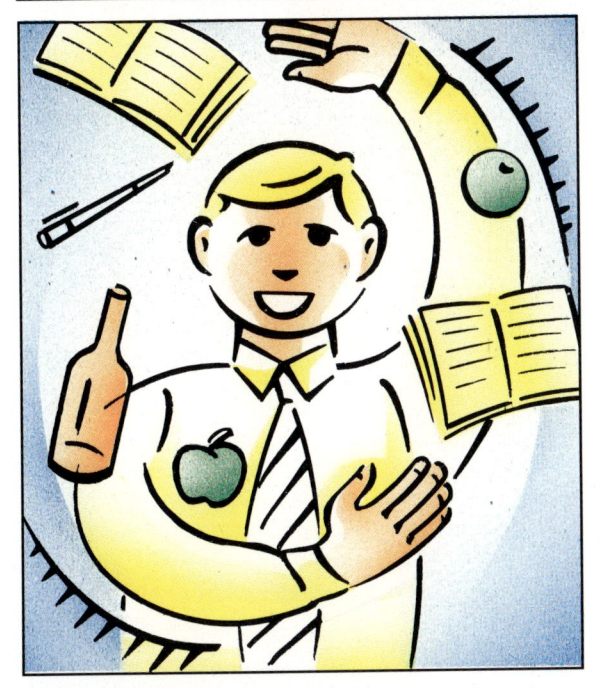

should have some solid food such as biscuits or sandwiches. If the child cannot take food he/she should be given one teaspoon of sugar in water or half a glass of lemonade every half hour until he/she can eat properly.

Children who have had a severe hypo may not feel well and could have a bad headache but they should be given sympathetic but firm encouragement to eat and drink.

If the child loses consciousness, is unable to swallow or simply will not take treatment, send for medical help. Remember: never give anything by mouth to an unconscious child as the food may be inhaled, leading to choking.

If the doctor is not in the immediate vicinity, it is better to call for an ambulance to take the child to the casualty section of the nearest hospital. Ambulance officers may also be able to administer injections of glucose or glucagon if necessary.

Glucagon is a hormone which makes the liver release stored sugar into the blood stream. All parents of children with diabetes should be able to give such an injection and should discuss with the doctor the right dosage. (See chapter 11 – Hypoglycaemia and Hyperglycaemia)

Generally for children aged under five, half the contents of the ampoule (0.5mg or unit) is given. For others, the whole ampoule is needed.

Giving such injections is a skill easily learnt and one which teachers should ideally acquire if taking children with diabetes on overnight excursions.

The effect of the glucagon is temporary and as soon as the child has recovered sufficiently, the usual treatment applies – a glass of lemonade or two heaped teaspoons of sugar in a glass of water, followed by solid food.

Preventing hypoglycaemia

The child with diabetes usually has two insulin injections a day. Once the insulin has been injected it lowers blood glucose until the insulin wears off. The glucose coming from food raises blood glucose. It is important for the child with diabetes to have meals at the same time each day.

It is especially important that the child with diabetes not miss meals or snacks.

Hypos occur most commonly just before meals are due and so the teacher will need to keep an unobtrusive eye on the child around this time. If there are any warning signs, food should be given immediately.

A second time when hypos frequently occur is during or after exercise and teachers supervising sport or exercise should be aware of this if there is a child with diabetes in their care.

The reason for the reaction to exercise is because muscles use more blood glucose when they are being used actively. The reaction will be different in different cases. Some children may have a hypo during exercise, some immediately afterwards and others not for hours later.

Therefore it is best to give extra food before exercise and also during any prolonged activities.

The best type of food is a mixture of rapidly absorbed sugar and a more slowly absorbed form. An ideal mix would be a drink of orange juice or sweet lemonade, an orange, or two or three lumps of sugar followed by starchy carbohydrates such as bread or plain, sweet biscuits.

A sandwich made with honey or jam would be suitable, or an energy bar – especially the type favoured by other children.

Ketoacidosis

A more serious problem for the child with diabetes is ketoacidosis which is associated with a high level of glucose in the blood and is a sign of a serious inadequacy of insulin.

It usually occurs during sick days when the child is unwell with severe colds, influenza and other feverish illnesses when the body requires extra insulin.

Ketoacidosis may also be caused by insulin injections being missed or the dose being too low.

Far less common than hypoglycaemia, ketoacidosis comes on gradually over hours or days and is marked by excessive urination and thirst and subsequent vomiting. It requires prompt medical attention.

For the teacher, the golden rules for diabetes are:
- If in doubt, give sugar. If the child is having a hypo, improvement will come over the next 15 minutes. If it is ketoacidosis, there will be no improvement.
- Should a child with diabetes commence vomiting, contact the parents or seek medical advice immediately.
- Never leave the child unattended and never let the sick child go home alone.

Food and diabetes

The young child with diabetes will usually bring a specially prepared lunch to school, but as the child grows older and becomes more knowledgeable, food may be bought from the school canteen.

There is nothing extraordinary about the diet. It is just a well balanced meal low in simple sugars.

However, food must be fairly constant in its quality and timing. The teacher is usually asked to ensure the meal is not skipped or delayed, and it would be useful for the canteen to stock low calorie soft drinks suitable for people with diabetes.

In general, extra food of any kind should only be given before exercise or to stop a hypo.

Psychological problems

The child with diabetes will have to contend with many pressures, from daily blood tests and injections to peer group pressure and uncertainty about the future, all of which may cause significant psychological problems.

In turn, this may make the diabetes less stable, adding to the pressures which must be faced.

There is much that can be done at school level to help the child overcome these problems.

For a start, every encouragement should be given to the child to join school activities to the full, be it sports, excursions or camps. *Remember, parents and teachers do the child no favours by singling them out for special attention and trying to shield them from what other children go through. People with diabetes excel in many fields, including sports.*

Bearing this in mind though, it is important to make certain allowances. For instance, the child with diabetes may require extra time to get ready for sport. There is food to be eaten, they may need a blood glucose test or may have to dispose of orange peel or sweet wrappings. All this should be taken into account by the teacher or sports supervisor. Sometimes the child with diabetes will need to eat between classes or during examinations.

Examinations may pose a special problem, especially if pre-exam nerves stop the child from eating the normal amount of food or if nervous tension burns up more than usual amounts of sugar.

Remember that a child having a hypo will not be able to think as well as usual. For the important senior examinations many school boards make allowances, such as allowing students with diabetes to eat during exams or leave to go to the toilet.

If a hypo did occur, extra time may have to be given to enable the student to perform to the best of their ability.

Childrens' Camps

These camps are a wonderful holiday for children as well as giving the parents a break. More importantly, however, the children have a good influence upon each other so that they undertake responsibilities which they previously refused eg: self-injecting. Regular diabetes camps are run in most States and Territories. Check with your local Diabetes Australia Association or The Juvenile Diabetes Foundation – Australia.

❏ ❏ ❏

To sum up

In all cases, communication between teachers, parents and child is the key.

It is a fine line between protecting the child and stifling natural potential. The child will require certain special treatment, but at the same time must not feel different from classmates.

With patience, empathy and communication, the school days of a child with diabetes can be just as rewarding and enlightening as for any other child.

CHAPTER 23

Diabetes – A Problem in Any Language

By Bernadette Lowther
Senior Diabetes Educator
Diabetes Australia –
New South Wales

Many of Australia's migrant communities suffer an increased risk of diabetes – greater not only than that of the existing population, but also of the risk they would have faced if they had remained in their country of origin.

Maltese, Maori, Greek and Tongan people are just some of the groups who are affected in this way. Researchers believe there are many factors for this, some to do with the new environment and some with a tendency towards diabetes which the migrants inherited.

In a similar way, Australian Aborigines have a greater risk of developing diabetes because of the change from their traditional lifestyle to a Western lifestyle. (See Chapter 24)

The problem of diabetes can be even greater than usual in these cases, with people who are not fluent in English finding it hard to learn about diabetes or acquaint themselves with the services available.

It is a two-way problem. The people with diabetes find it difficult to learn about their condition, while the health care workers find it hard to communicate with them.

It is important that the person with diabetes understands that in Australia everyone is entitled to an equal share of the health care system, regardless of their cultural background.

Likewise, it is essential that health

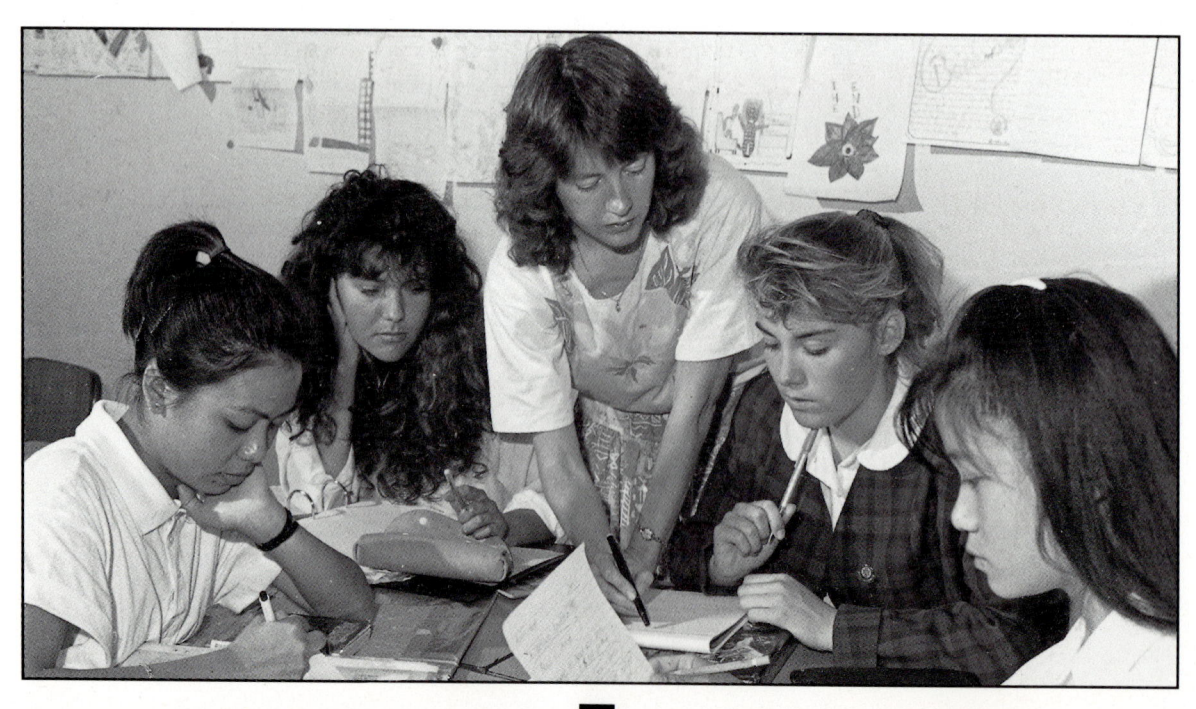

professionals appreciate the cultural characteristics of the individual and tailor information and treatment to suit.

It is the right of any person to have an interpreter present, if necessary, when being seen by a health professional. The health worker should be notified in advance if an interpreter is required.

In Australia there are many services for the person with diabetes, and it is important to know just what is available to ensure the best possible treatment.

For this reason, it is a good idea to put together a list of all available resources under three categories: People, Material Resources and Existing Facilities.

People

This could be divided into two sections, Health Professionals and Community Workers.

Under Health Professionals list doctor, educator, dietitian, podiatrist, eye specialist, psychologist and occupational health officer.

Under Community Workers would come migrant health workers, interpreters and social workers.

Material Resources

The next category is Material Resources. There are written materials, video tapes and audio tapes about diabetes available in many languages. Diabetes Australia and your nearest Diabetes Education Centre will help you find what is available.

The most widely used book, currently available in 10 languages, is "Diabetes – What You Need To Know" and may be obtained by contacting Diabetes Australia.

In the near future Diabetes Australia will be producing a range of education materials in several different languages for national distribution.

Existing Facilities

Locally, you should list the nearest Diabetes Education Centres (which are usually attached to hospitals or community centres), hospital-based outpatients clinics, to which your doctor can refer you, and Community health Centres.

Each State or Territory has a range of migrant health services including telephone interpreters and education materials. These organisations are listed in the telephone directory.

On a national basis organisations such as Diabetes Australia and Juvenile Diabetes Foundation – Australia can provide useful information.

There are also government subsidised products, such as blood and urine testing strips and syringes, which are available. To qualify for the subsidy it is necessary to register at a Diabetes Australia office.

❏ ❏ ❏

For further information about the many services available, refer to the chapter 28 *Further Resources* **in this book.**

CHAPTER 24

Diabetes in Aborigines

By Professor Kerin O'Dea
Professor of Nutrition
Deakin University
Melbourne

There is no evidence that diabetes or other lifestyle diseases such as obesity, cardiovascular disease or hypertension occurred among Aborigines when they lived traditionally.

Most Aborigines today lead a westernised lifestyle, with a diet based on western foods and with sedentary, physically inactive lives.

Under these circumstances many become overweight and develop Type 2 diabetes.

Diabetes is common enough among white Australians, with 3.4 per cent contracting the condition, but in most urbanised Aboriginal communities the prevalence is much greater, ranging from as low as 5 per cent in the least westernised communities, to as high as 24 per cent in the most westernised, overweight communities.

In many Aboriginal communities over half the people aged over 40 have either diabetes or impaired glucose tolerance. There is also evidence of greater risk of cardiovascular disease in these communities, as well as hypertension, hyperlipidemia, ECG abnormalities and high insulin levels which is consistent with insulin resistance.

The public health implications of these high rates of diabetes are enormous. People with diabetes are at higher risk for coronary heart disease, stroke, peripheral vascular disease, gangrene, skin infections, renal failure and peripheral neuropathy.

The public health implications are even more serious when it is considered that many Aborigines are contracting diabetes in their early 20s and 30s and the younger they are, the greater the risk of complications.

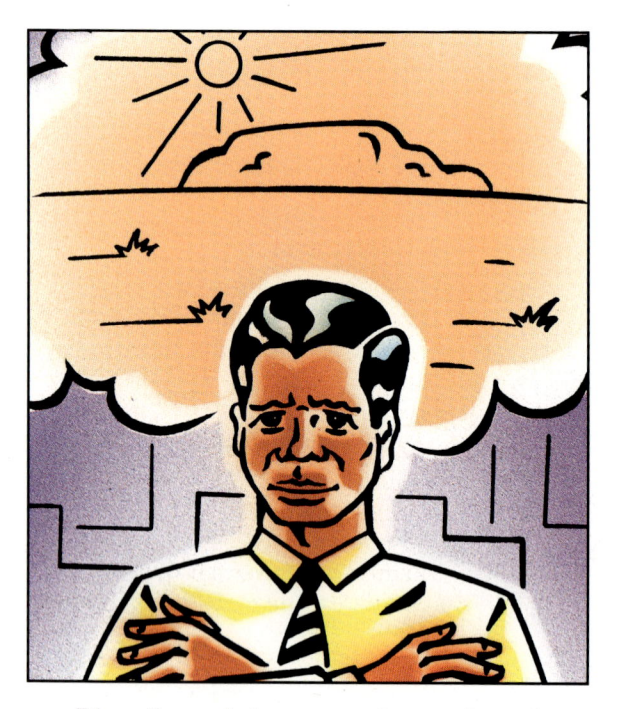

The financial costs of treating these conditions are increasing sharply, not to mention the personal costs in terms of loss of quality of life.

Diabetes in Aborigines has failed to respond to conventional therapies for a number of cultural, historic and economic reasons. Innovative strategies are therefore essential if the epidemic is to be controlled.

So Why are Aborigines so vulnerable to diabetes?

The type of diabetes occurring among Aborigines is Type 2 diabetes, the predominant form among white Australians.

As explained in Types of Diabetes (Chapter 2) this type of diabetes develops as a consequence of genetic susceptibility being triggered by certain lifestyle factors.

The precise nature of the genetic susceptibility is not well understood but it is believed resistance to the action of insulin may be the main factor.

Therefore any aspect of lifestyle which worsens insulin resistance could act as a trigger to precipitate the disease.

It is probably no coincidence that lack of exercise, obesity, an energy dense diet rich in fat and sugar and depleted of fibre, plus excessive energy intake, are known to worsen insulin resistance and are also recognised as risk factors for Type 2 diabetes.

In the case of the Aborigines, it is likely that their traditional hunter-gatherer lifestyle protected them against Type 2 diabetes by maximising insulin sensitivity.

As nomadic hunter-gatherers they were extremely lean and physically fit. Their diet was derived from wild animals, fish and uncultivated vegetables.

This diet was bulky, with a low energy density. Wild animals and fish have a very low fat content and the uncultivated vegetables were high in fibre, vitamins and essential trace metals, as well as containing carbohydrates which were slowly digested and absorbed.

In fact, the traditional diet had all the qualities now recognised as important in the treatment and prevention of Type 2 diabetes: high fibre, low fat, slowly digested carbohydrate. All coupled with a high level of physical activity and extreme leanness to maximise insulin sensitivity.

With the change to a western lifestyle, physical activity declined dramatically and the diet changed greatly: out went the fibre, and in came increased energy intake of sugar, fat and alcohol.

The efficient metabolism, once a survival mechanism now promotes overweight, diabetes and the associated conditions of hypertension and cardiovascular disease.

It is possible that all these conditions share a common pathway: insulin resistance – increased by such a change in lifestyle.

Reversing the process

So the question must be asked: if lifestyle change causes diabetes in Aborigines, can it be treated by reversing the process?

This was the idea behind a study in 1982, when 14 Aborigines from a remote community in WA – ten with diabetes, and four without, participated in a study which saw them revert to the traditional lifestyle.

Metabolic tests were conducted before and after seven weeks of living off the land.

The results were striking, with a marked improvement in all the metabolic abnormalities of diabetes, plus a reduction in a number of risk factors for cardiovascular disease.

As far as the abnormalities of diabetes were concerned, some, such as high plasma triglycerides, were completely normalised while others, such as fasting glucose, glucose tolerance and insulin secretion were not, although they improved greatly.

Had the study continued longer they may have been corrected. As it was, seven weeks of traditional lifestyle were enough to substantially reverse a disease which took years to develop in the urban environment.

The public health implications are enormous. Not only is diabetes potentially reversible in Aborigines, but potentially preventable as well.

The results of the study are a dramatic illustration of the relationship between lifestyle and health. There were three major components of traditional lifestyle which would have contributed to the improved metabolic control – regular physical activity, low fat, high fibre diet and weight loss.

These three factors are all a natural part of the hunter-gatherer lifestyle and in the urban context all have to be addressed separately.

- Increased physical activity: ideally this should be incorporated in the daily routine, such as walking rather than driving, carrying out manual labour or taking part in sport. This represents a major philosophical shift for the hunter-gatherer who in the traditional lifestyle

would have minimised "unnecessary" energy output in the interests of efficiency.
- Low fat, high fibre diet. A key component for many communities is their local general store, where all too frequently health takes second place to short-term profit in determining the type of foods sold. However, health and profit do not have to be opposed and there are examples of financially profitable stores in Aboriginal communities which stock high quality food and promote the consumption of fruit, vegetables, wholegrain cereals, lean meats, low fat dairy products and the like. Unfortunately such successes are few and have depended on intensive input from public health professionals such as nutritionists.
- Weight loss in the overweight. If the first two components are implemented, the third should follow automatically.

The epidemic of lifestyle diseases such as diabetes in Aboriginal communities justifies the development of community-wide programs aimed at treatment and prevention.

Prevention is better than cure and the cluster of lifestyle diseases such as obesity, diabetes, hypertension, cardiovascular disease and hyperlipidemias will all respond to changes in diet and exercise.

The challenge for Aborigines is to devise appropriate strategies to encourage healthpromoting change and the key is that such programmes be designed and run by Aborigines.

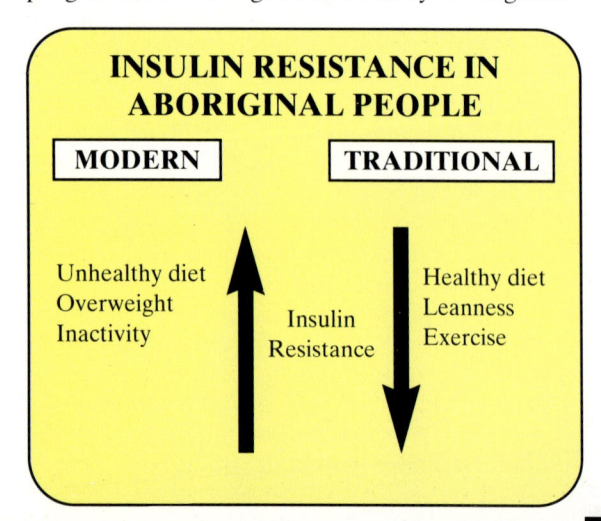

Unless Aborigines "own" such programs, it is unlikely they will be taken up over the long term. The success of the "back-to-the-bush" study was probably due in part to its "Aboriginality".

The benefits went far beyond the physical health of the participants, their self esteem also increased enormously. People considered failures in town, such as alcoholics, were capable, successful hunters in the bush.

The strong links these people had with their land and the renewal evident when they returned to it was very moving and highlighted the potentially important relationship between landrights and health.

Probably the most important implication to be drawn from the association between diabetes and the westernisation of Aborigines is the very real potential for prevention of Type 2 diabetes.

This is particularly relevant for the children and other close relatives of people with diabetes.

One of the best predictors of susceptibility to Type 2 diabetes is a family history of the disease. The stronger the family history, the greater the risk.

However this genetic susceptibility need not be taken as a foregone conclusion. Aborigines did not get diabetes when they lived traditionally and the principles of that lifestyle could be applied to protect the offspring of people with diabetes.

As all people with diabetes are only too aware, prevention is clearly preferable to treatment and it is theoretically possible in most cases.

Unfortunately by the time many people are diagnosed as having Type 2 diabetes the condition is well established and intervention to reverse the process is more difficult.

The implications for white people with Type 2 diabetes

The same principles inherent in the hunter-gatherer lifestyle can be applied to the treatment of Type 2 diabetes generally.

Regular physical activity, a low fat, high fibre diet and weight loss remain the cornerstone of therapy for the vast majority of people with Type 2 diabetes.

INSULIN RESISTANCE IN ABORIGINAL PEOPLE

MODERN	TRADITIONAL
Unhealthy diet Overweight Inactivity ↑	Healthy diet Leanness Exercise ↓

Insulin Resistance

All of these factors have been shown to be independently effective in improving metabolic control in Type 2 diabetes with the underlying mechanism of effectiveness apparently related to improved sensitivity to insulin.

As was also evident with the bush study, these lifestyle changes have numerous other beneficial health consequences, not the least of which is improved self-confidence. Accordingly, the importance of the person with diabetes taking control of their treatment cannot be overstressed.

Since Type 2 diabetes is a condition brought on by lifestyle factors it stands to reason that the most rational approach to its treatment is through lifestyle modification.

It should be stressed however that such an approach will not work for all people with non-insulin dependent diabetes.

It is particularly appropriate for those with insulin resistance. Diabetic control in those with Type 2 diabetes in whom insulin resistance is not a major feature, may not be improved greatly by lifestyle modification.

Nevertheless, such a program would have general benefits in terms of modification of cardiovascular disease risk factors and could be combined with other therapy.

Type 2 diabetes is different from Type 1 diabetes – it is a symptomless condition in the early stages, often for years. Frequently it is picked up only by chance or as a result of the development of complications.

Intervention based on lifestyle modification is most effective in the early stages when the major metabolic abnormalities appear to be reversible.

❏ ❏ ❏

It has been argued convincingly that the hunter-gatherer diet and lifestyle is what we are geneticaly programmed for – that it has been the lifestyle of humans for the greater part of their history. If so, it makes a lot of sense to go back to that diet and lifestyle in our search for solutions to many of our current health problems. And if successful, the principles of such a solution will undoubtedly have wider application than simply in prevention and treatment of Type 2 diabetes.

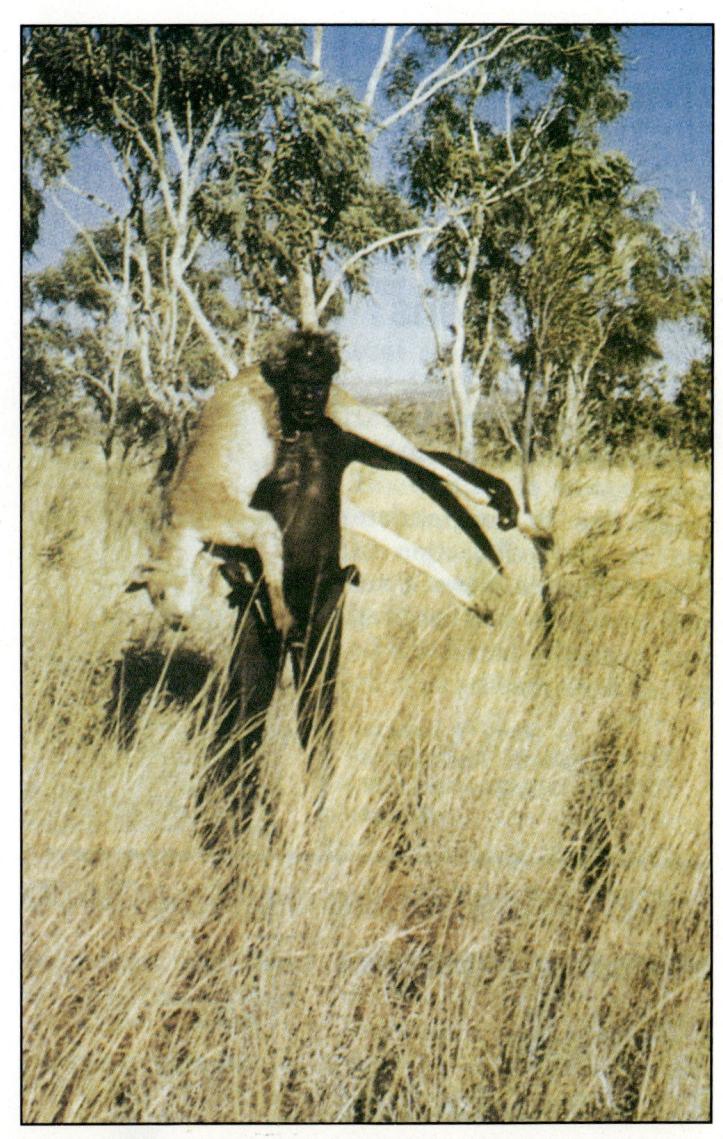

When a group of Aborigines return to their traditional lifestyle control of diabetes improved dramatically.

DIABETES & YOU
An owner's manual

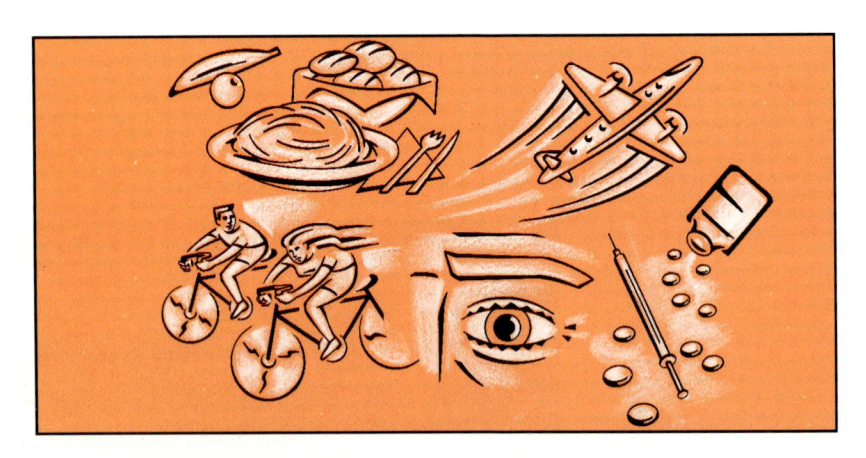

SOCIAL ISSUES

❏ **Rights and Responsibilities**
   Your rights
   What you need to know
   Steps to better control of diabetes
   What your doctor will check

❏ **Insurance and Diabetes**
   Good news
   The company's view
   Information required
   The official policy
   Influencing factors
   Advice on insurance
   Superannuation

❏ **Travel**
   Essential preliminary preparation
   Your itinerary
   Personal documents
   Luggage
   Food en route
   When you arrive
   Insulin
   Insulin dosage
   Jet lag
   Sick days
   Blood and urine testing
   Medications
   Motion sickness

❏ **Further Resources**
   Diabetes Australia – a good place to start
   Hospitals, Clinics and Community Centres
   Doctors
   Other Health Professionals
   Bookshops and libraries
   Where to look for help

Rights and Responsibilities

By David Nathan
Ex President
Juvenile Diabetes Foundation Australia
Sydney

People with diabetes are in essence no different from any other members of the community. They have rights and they have responsibilities.

For instance, they have the right of access to the treatment, education and support services to enable them to best control their diabetes. They have the responsibility for themselves – they must take charge of their treatment to ensure successful management of their condition.

Your rights

Like anyone else, you have rights.
If you wish, you are entitled to:
- Professional health services, appropriate medication and glucose testing strips and meters.
- A clear understandable explanation about your condition and a sympathetic hearing and discussion with the health professional who will provide any necessary treatment or investigations. If necessary interpreter services should be made available.
- Access to diabetes literature, education and educators.
- Access to specialist physicians, eye specialists, dietitians and podiatrists and other specialists as necessary.
- A second opinion about your treatment.
- The career of your choice, life and health insurance cover, job training or appropriate civil licenses and permits. If these are denied, contact your specialist who will determine if exclusion is justified.
- Specialised care of your diabetes when in hospital for other conditions.
- Continue your own insulin injections and carry out your own blood glucose tests when in hospital.

And finally, remember – you have the right to the last say.

What you need to know

It must always be remembered that the responsibility for control of your diabetes ultimately rests with you. You will be advised and monitored by your doctor, but when all is said and done, regular procedures such as dieting, testing, exercising, taking medications properly, footcare and coping with high or low blood sugars are up to you.

In some instances of course the responsibility must be shared or delegated. In the case of a young child, the aged, infirm or mentally handicapped for instance, relatives or other people will have to step in and take charge.

In the majority of cases though reasonable standards of care and delegation of responsibilities should be achieved by the people with diabetes themselves.

Diabetes is never mild. Even those on diet alone can develop complications. Prolonged poor control makes the chances of damage to eyesight, kidneys, sexual potency, blood flow to heart, brain and legs all more likely.

But whether there is some damage to your body or not, much can be done to prevent problems.

Some of the steps to better control of diabetes

- Become as fully informed as possible about your condition. Contact Diabetes Australia or the Juvenile Diabetes Foundation Australia for extra information. Seek out and attend diabetes education courses at your local hospital, health centre or diabetes education

centre. Ask questions until you are comfortable with the answers.
- Ask your general practitioner to refer you to a dietitian and obtain a meal plan. This should be done at the time of diagnosis, and at regular intervals afterwards.
- Ask for referral to a specialist experienced in diabetes care before commencing insulin injections.
- If you are planning to become pregnant, see a diabetes specialist before stopping contraception. If you are already pregnant you will need urgent referral and on-going care from an expert throughout the pregnancy.
- If you are controlled by diet or diet and tablet treatment, you may be referred to a specialist if problems arise.
- Use any time with a specialist as a further step in your education process. Ask questions and follow any advice.
- Identify those factors which alter control. Stop smoking, cut down on alcohol, exercise regularly after checking with your doctor, shed excess weight.
- See a dietitian and eat a healthy diet – cutting down on fats and increasing vegetables, fruit and cereals.
- Test blood or urine glucose levels and record the results accurately to enable your doctor to make the right decision concerning your treatment.
- Learn what to expect when you visit the general practitioner or specialist.

What your doctor will check

Eyes (See chapter 16)

If you are under 30 you should see an eye specialist after five years of diabetes and at intervals as advised.

If you are over 30 you should see a specialist at the time of diagnosis and then as advised.

Remember, serious eye damage may be developing even though your eyesight is still excellent. Early detection means better treatment and blindness can be prevented – but not reversed.

Blood Pressure

High blood pressure may worsen any damage caused by diabetes to your kidneys, heart, circulation and eyes. Treatment of high blood pressure can prevent these problems.

Feet (See chapter 17)

Diabetes can damage the circulation and sensation in your feet, making them susceptible to damage. This is why your doctor will regularly check the skin, pulses and sensation in your feet. Make it easy for the doctor by dressing appropriately.

Weight and Height

Excess weight makes diabetic control difficult and it contributes to poor blood glucose control, high cholesterol, high blood pressure and heart disease.

Because of this your doctor will weigh you regularly to assess your progress. If you are still growing he will also measure your height as growth may be stunted by poor glucose control.

Insulin Injection Sites

These will be checked regularly by the doctor because problems at these sites can worsen your control.

Pathology Tests

Become interested in the pathology tests ordered by your doctor. The common ones are:
- Glycated Haemoglobin – usually done several times a year. It shows what your overall blood glucose control has been over the previous two or three months. An alternative test is fructosamine which measures your overall control over the previous two or three weeks.
- Cholesterol, Triglycerides and High Density Lipoprotein are important blood fats that the doctor usually measures every year. High cholesterol seems an important cause of heart attack and circulation problems. A healthy eating pattern, with or without certain medications, can reduce high cholesterol levels.
- Creatinine is a test of kidney function usually carried out once a year.

Rights and Responsibilities

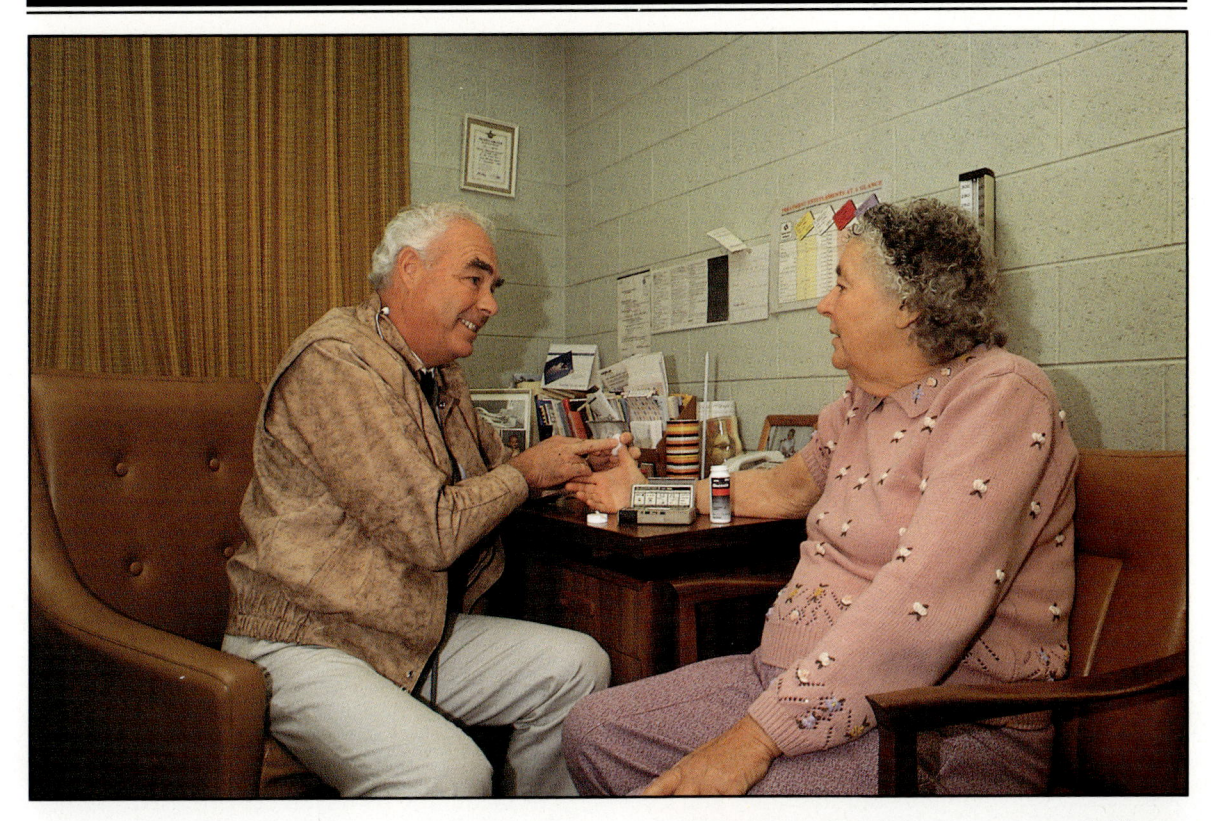

– Microalbuminuria – a test on urine that may be carried out to detect early kidney damage due to diabetes.

❏ ❏ ❏

Remember that it is your responsibility to manage your diabetes and your right to access the resources you need.

CHAPTER 26

Insurance and Diabetes

By Dr John Carter
Consultant Endocrinologist
Hornsby and Ku-ring-gai Hospital
and Concord Hospital
Sydney

To most people life insurance is a case of picking up the telephone and choosing the lowest premium. For people with diabetes, it is not that simple.

For many years there have been concerns within the diabetes community over the expense and hassles associated with obtaining life insurance.

Insurance is not always easy to get, and when it is granted, the premium is considerably higher than for other people.

To a certain degree this must be expected, but many people with diabetes believe the statistics used by the insurance industry to justify these increased premiums are outdated and do not reflect the benefits of modern diabetes management.

Good news

There is no question that regular breakthroughs in the treatment of diabetes have led to greatly improved quality of life and increased life-span but still some people are being denied insurance and others are charged annual premiums which they believe are unfair.

The good news is that improved life expectancy figures and consumer pressure are having an effect and many Australian companies are changing their outlook, although not as quickly as in other countries.

In Denmark for instance, extensive studies

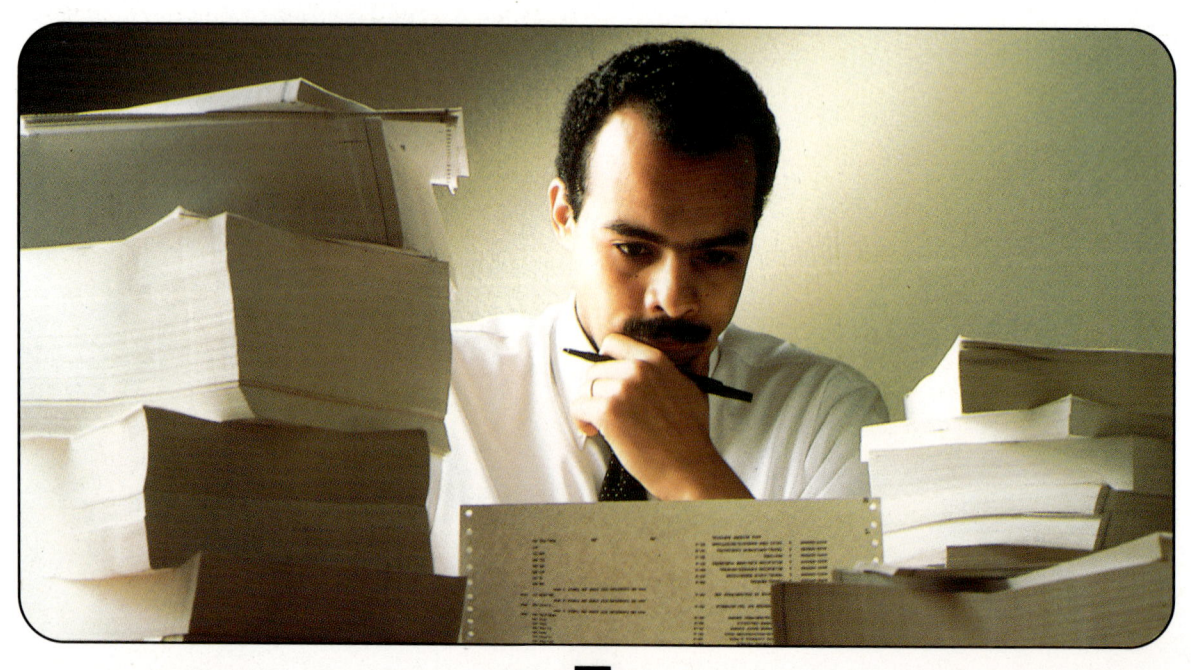

have been carried out clearly documenting the improvements in quality of lifestyle and life span for people with diabetes over the past 50 years.

The figures show that people with Type I diabetes have experienced a 15 to 30 year increase in life expectancy.

The findings have been accepted by the insurance industry in Denmark and passed on to the diabetic community accordingly.

The attitude in Australia is not so enlightened but progress is being made.

The Company's view

It is important to realise that offering insurance to people with diabetes presents difficulties for the underwriter.

This is because diabetes is not a single disorder and represents a wide group of disorders with disturbed metabolism of glucose as the common factor. Just as there is no fixed definition of "diabetes", there is no fixed rule when it comes to insurance.

For this reason it is unusual for pure life insurance – that is, insurance with the sum insured being payable on death or on survival to a specified date, to be turned down solely because of the proposer's diabetes.

Usually cover can be offered on some grounds.

Information required

Before final assessment of the proposal, the insurance company will require comprehensive medical information, consisting of:
- A diabetic questionnaire regarding history and management of the condition
- A detailed report from the person's doctor, including the date of diagnosis, type of diabetes, nature of treatment and response to treatment.
- Report on a current medical examination

For larger policies, the company will require more comprehensive medical information.

The underwriter would take particular note if the medical information showed:
- Childhood onset of diabetes
- Duration of diabetes of less than one year since diagnosis
- Poor control of the condition
- Poor self-management of the condition
- Any existing diabetes-related complications
- Additional medical or lifestyle risks
- Inadequate documentation of medical history

The assessment rating would become even more severe – and perhaps even result in the proposal being turned down, if there were further complicating factors, such as:

> **COMPLICATING FACTORS**
> - Evidence of kidney disease, particularly if large amounts of protein were detected in the urine
> - Evidence of diabetic retinopathy
> - High blood pressure
> - Heart disease
> - Excessive alcohol intake
> - Smoking
> - Obesity
> - Evidence of peripheral neuropathy
> - Unfavourable family history, particularly relating to early deaths from heart and kidney disease.

For adults with diabetes the best terms are offered if diabetes is of short duration, such as less than ten years – as long as there are none of the unfavourable factors already mentioned.

Generally speaking, the later the age of onset, the more favourably the company will look on the proposal.

Insurance premiums generally increase with age, also advancing age often gives rise to other medical complications which may further limit availability of insurance. Because of this it is important to purchase insurance early.

The official policy

The Life Insurance Federation of Australia states that the terms offered to people with diabetes – as with everyone else, are based on available statistical evidence supplemented by the considered judgement of medical experts, underwriters and actuaries.

Each proposal is treated strictly on its merits and in accordance with the underwriting policy of the company concerned after consideration of evidence gathered at the time.

Insurance and Diabetes

Each company could differ to some degree in its ratings although the assessment criteria would generally not vary.

One company states "it needs to be borne in mind that it takes some time for both favourable and unfavourable developments in treatment, diagnosis, survival rates etc to be reflected in the Terms offered."

In addition, it should be emphasised that underwriting rules represent only part of the underwriting process and the differences in policy and competitive factors will often result in different offers being made from different insurance companies on proposals for the same person with diabetes.

Taking all this into consideration, it could be said that insurance cover for people with diabetes is generally available in Australia and that the terms offered will vary according to a number of criteria.

There is no reason to expect that an otherwise healthy person with well controlled diabetes could not be insured – albeit with significantly increased premiums.

Influencing factors

There are however factors which influence premiums over which people with diabetes have significant control:

FACTORS INFLUENCING PREMIUMS
- Excessive alcohol intake
- Smoking
- Control of blood pressure
- Obesity
- Conscientiousness with respect to management of diabetes
- Presence of any additional medical or lifestyle risks

Also, the person with diabetes hoping to take out an insurance policy should make certain their doctor knows the importance of them demonstrating good diabetic control and a freedom from the complications of diabetes. The doctor should also be made aware of just how important the medical report prepared for the insurance company is. Poorly presented medical evidence will undoubtedly result in a higher premium.

Advice on insurance

Advances in treatment are continually taking place in Australia and Diabetes Australia is actively lobbying insurance companies, keeping them informed of the latest data relating to improvements in quality of life and life-span.

In addition, there is increased competition in the marketplace and Diabetes Australia can supply advice on insurance policies currently available.

People with diabetes or at risk of contracting diabetes should get insurance as soon as possible and those with diabetes should at least look at the possibility of obtaining job positions which include group insurance or join groups which might give them more favourable consideration.

If in doubt about life assurance, sickness, accident or travel insurance, ask Diabetes Australia for advice.

Superannuation

Superannuation can be regarded as an investment whereby a lump sum or pension or combination of the two will be paid upon retirement. People retiring early, say for medical reasons, receive a lower benefit.

This investment component is not specifically affected by the presence of diabetes but many superannuation policies also include life insurance and/or disability insurance. Obviously factors outlined earlier would influence this type of policy.

Some work situations have automatic superannuation/life insurance/disability insurance cover. This may be advantageous for a person with diabetes as the regular superannuation contributions would include the insurance premiums -- without any loading.

As such it would be prudent to take superannuation into account, and study the fine print carefully, when considering a new job.

CHAPTER 27

Travel

By Clinical Associate Professor Paul Moffitt
Royal Newcastle Hospital
Newcastle

Ten years ago travelling overseas or through remote areas of Australia presented problems but now there is virtually no limit to where the person with diabetes can go.

The change has been brought about by a number of factors, such as: the ability of the person with diabetes to measure his or her own blood glucose level; patient and medical practitioner education and the greater understanding of diabetes it fosters; the availability of glucagon for injection; improved travel facilities and a worldwide public recognition of diabetes.

Regardless of the age of the traveller, the destination or the mode of transport, the preparation and travelling routine will be similar for all people with diabetes.

Preparation is of course a vitally important part of any trip, but even more so for the person with diabetes. The key is to prepare lists of things to do and take.

Essential preliminary preparations

The first list should be of essential preparations which cannot be left until the last minute. Included would be enquiries about health problems in the countries to be visited, vaccinations, renewing passport and names and addresses of diabetes services.

This early preparation should also include an approach to the local high school or relevant foreign consulate requesting a written translation of some essential phrases such as "I have diabetes" or "I have diabetes. Could you please quickly give me some sugar or something to eat."

Every person with diabetes should carry some form of identification, such as a bracelet, locket or less desirably, a card stating that the carrier has diabetes and requires certain medications. This is even more important when travelling and should be obtained long before departure – ask Diabetes Australia or your local Diabetes Education Centre.

Insurance

Medicare is not responsible for health expenses incurred overseas and you would not believe how costly these may be. Suppose your passport, tickets, traveller's cheques, credit cards or luggage are stolen – what will you do? The answer is that Travel Insurance is cheap and is as essential as your fares. Ask your travel agent or Diabetes Australia.

Your itinerary

Another item would be a reminder to direct the travel agent to obtain an accurate itinerary of your trip with departure and arrival times, duration of flight sections, stopovers and approximate meal or snack times. See chart 1 on page 126.

It is really only insulin requiring people with diabetes who need this information but it is essential for safe and intelligent insulin administration – therefore do not accept the excuse that such information is not available. This is also the opportunity for you to notify the airline of any special requirements which you or your child or infant with diabetes may require.

Personal documents

Personal documents could be the heading for another list which could include Australian and foreign currency, travellers' cheques, passport, air tickets, health certificate, international credit

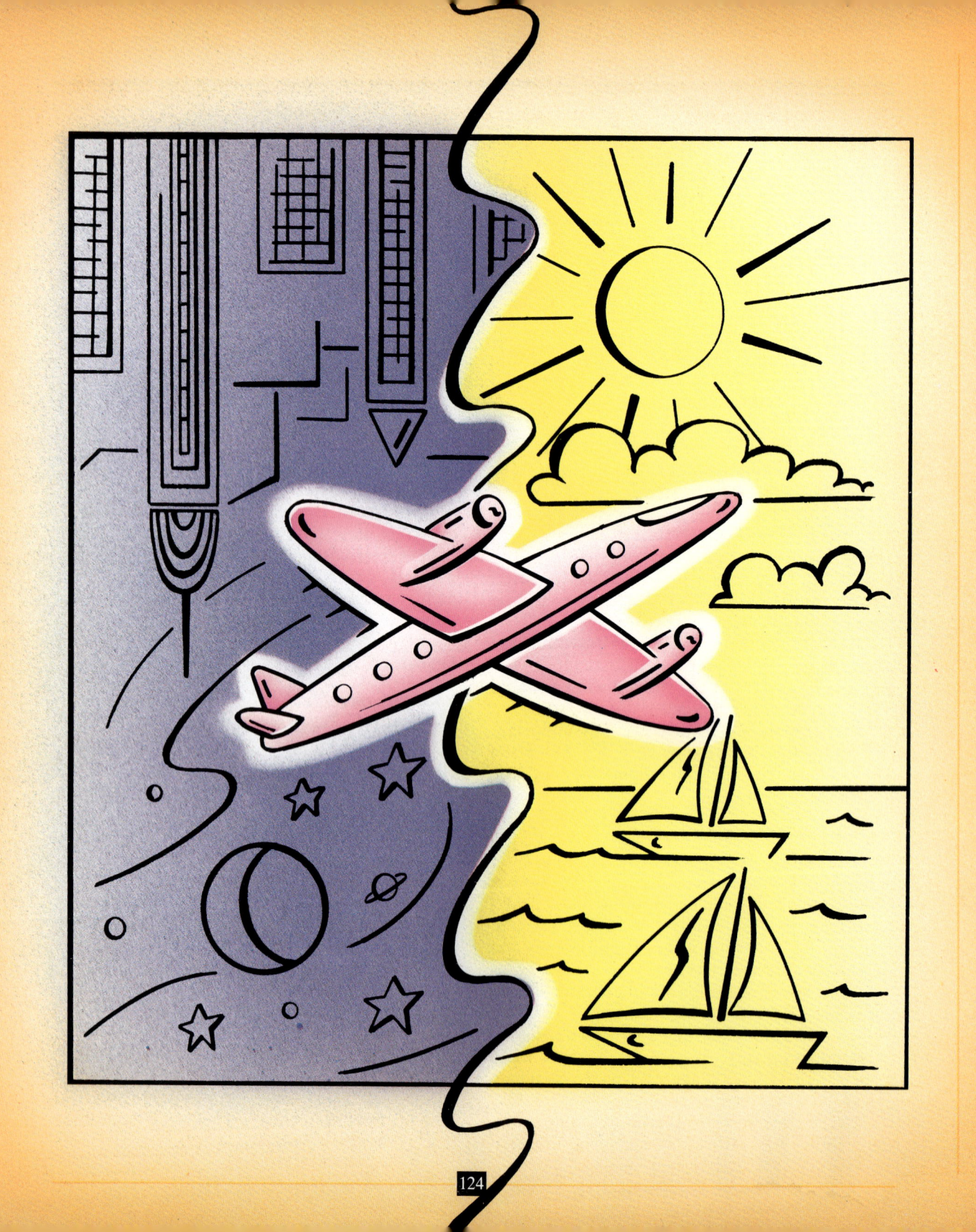

card, addresses of contacts, letter from doctor, details of itinerary. These items are all essential and should be carried in such a way that theft is almost impossible. Neglect this, and your trip may be ruined.

Hand luggage

No matter what mode of transport you take, or whether in Australia or overseas, you will require hand luggage and you must therefore prepare a list. You should take twice as many medications as are required and they should be divided into equal halves shared between your hand luggage and that of your travelling companion. If you are travelling alone your medications should be distributed equally between your hand luggage and stowed luggage.

Other luggage

Obviously a further list is required for your major luggage and possibly yet another if your trip includes another element such as trekking or canoeing.

Food en route

International flights usually offer an over abundance of food but this does not mean food will be available when you require it. It is therefore essential to carry extra carbohydrate in your hand luggage no matter what your mode of transport.

As any traveller will attest, no matter what form of transport you take, delays are a fact of life. Therefore, be prepared – carry food with you on and off planes, buses or cars.

This is equally important for people with Type 2 diabetes as tablets can produce hypoglycaemia and unconsciousness if a meal is missed.

Airlines can supply diabetic diets if notified at least 48 hours prior to departure. This will ensure not only that you will have the correct food, but that the flight staff are aware you have diabetes.

It is possible, but not certain, that your meals will be served prior to that of the other passengers but this is of no real advantage unless you require food quickly and have specifically asked to be served first.

Remember, you should not expect the airline to roll out the red carpet just because you have diabetes, so do not ask for unnecessary services such as meals outside the scheduled times. However a request for extra carbohydrate between meals would be rarely refused particularly if the traveller is carrying a letter from a medical practitioner. (See Chart on page 131)

Once again though, as we have stressed throughout this book, the key is to take control of your own condition and be prepared for whatever might occur.

> *For instance, there is the case of the Australian on a domestic flight in the US who started suffering symptoms of a hypo. Unprepared, he called the flight attendant, informed her he had diabetes and asked for sugar. She refused until it could be approved by a doctor.*
>
> *A doctor on the flight answered the call but he too refused permission until the patient had undertaken a urine test. Sugar was then denied because there was sugar in the urine.*
>
> *The man suffered severe hypoglycaemia and unconsciousness and spent three days in hospital. Because he was unprepared, he suffered a great deal of discomfort and spent a lot of money - when half a dozen jelly beans in his hand luggage would have sufficed.*

When you arrive

One of the joys of travelling is to eat the food of the country one is visiting but this must be done with discretion in some countries. The scenery might be a delight, but the diarrhoea which comes after drinking the water, milk or fluid in an unsealed bottle, or eating uncooked vegetables or unpeeled fruit is definitely not.

Mineral water bottled by reputable firms can be purchased in most countries, however despite the utmost diligence it must be expected that one of your party, maybe you yourself, will get traveller's diarrhoea and you should be prepared. This will be covered later in the chapter.

Travel

Frank Harris

	am	pm
Actrapid	14	6
Monotard	36	16

HOME TIME	AIRPORT	LOCAL TIME ARR. DEP.	DURATION	FROM DEPARTURE TO MEAL SNACK	INSULIN	OTHER*
1545	SYDNEY	1545	9½ hrs		Actrapid 4 Monotard 12	Blood Test
1700						
1800				—		Blood Test
1900				2 hrs		
2000				—		
2100						
2200				—		
2300						Blood Test
2400						
0100	BANGKOK	1015				
0200	BANGKOK		1¼ hrs			Walk Around
0300	BANGKOK	1130	12 hr 25 min	—		Blood Test
0400				¾ hr		
0500				—	AT BANGKOK AIRPORT	
0600						
0700				—		
0800						Blood Test
0900				—		
1000					Actrapid 6–10	Blood Test
1100				—		
1200						
1300				—		Blood Test
1400				11 hrs	Actrapid 6 Monotard 36	
1500				—		
1600	LONDON	0555				Blood Test

* After arrival in London take additional Actrapid between 1100 and 1400 hours, if necessary, then normal evening dosage. Blood glucose levels under 7 mmol/l require extra food. Meals and snacks listed are those provided by the airline.

(CHART 1)

Travel

Insulin

As already stated, insulin should be divided equally with half in your hand luggage, half in your travelling companion's hand luggage. If this is not possible half may have to go in your stowed luggage.

This is not ideal because the baggage of some aircraft may, on occasions, reach freezing point and this will destroy your insulin.

It is highly unlikely that this could occur on a large, international airline but it is possible with some older or smaller aircraft on long flights. Insulin which has frozen and thawed will look no different to the untrained eye so there is no method of telling whether it has been frozen or not.

To reduce the likelihood of insulin being frozen, it should be packed in a polystyrene container and further insulated by being wrapped in clothing and placed in the centre of the suitcase.

Heat will also destroy insulin, so as well as being carried in a polystyrene container, it should never be left in places such as the glove box, trunk or roof rack of a motor vehicle, in outside pockets of back-packs or near heat sources such as engines.

Strips are available to indicate temperature changes between 37°C and 65°C. These strips and your insulin should be placed together in the coolest part of your baggage.

When travelling by air in some countries in which your baggage could be subjected to high temperatures on the tarmac or freezing temperatures in an aircraft's hold, one of these strips should be included with your insulin in your stowed luggage.

Insulin is not affected by the x-ray equipment used at airports to scan luggage.

All insulin used in Australia and New Zealand is 100 units per ml. This is also available in Great Britain, the US and many other countries, although in some areas only weaker insulins may be available.

If forced to buy these *weaker* insulins – 40 units/ml or 80 units/ml, it is desirable to buy the correct syringe at the same time. You would then use your own dosage with that syringe.

Do not purchase a syringe that does not have a marking on it identifying it as being designed for U40 or U80 insulin.

If in doubt it would be wiser to use your own unit 100 syringes and adjust the dosage accordingly. U40 insulin used in your U100 syringe would require two and a half times as much fluid as your U100 strength insulin. For example a dosage of 30 units of U40 needs 30 x 2½ = the equivalent of 75 units in your U100 syringe. Using U80 insulin in your U100 syringe requires 1¼ times the usual dose and therefore 30 x 1¼ = the equivalent of 37½ units in your U100 syringe.

The insulin used in an insulin pen in Australia is also U100 and can be used in an ordinary U100 syringe if the pen is broken, lost or stolen. The insulin is extracted from the pen cartridge without injecting the correct amount of air prior to extracting the desired dosage of insulin. So don't forget to take an ordinary syringe as well as your pen.

Insulin dosage

Insulin dosage should not be of concern during travel unless there has been or will be a marked change in exercise or diet. Any rapid change in time zone as you travel will also have an effect. Any change in diet should have been anticipated and prepared for through consultation with your doctor or dietitian. It may also be wise to experiment with some of the anticipated dishes before you leave.

Major changes in exercise have been covered in Chapter 12, Diabetes and Exercise, and are unlikely to occur except with people who are experienced in such changes. The basic rule is that if prolonged exercise is to be undertaken the person with diabetes should either increase the carbohydrate of the diet preceding, during and after the exercise and/or reduce the insulin dosage prior to exercise. This would really be a matter of judgement based on experience.

Air flights in a northerly or southerly direction do not result in significant time changes and should not interfere with insulin dosage. Flights in an easterly or westerly direction, depending on their duration, may result in substantial changes which must be considered when adjusting insulin dosage.

The problem is that the person flying east is flying in the opposite direction to the passage of the sun, and therefore shortening the day. In other words, if that person had stayed in Sydney it could have been evening meal time at 6pm, with the next day's pre-breakfast insulin 13 hours away. If that person had flown to say Los Angeles though, the time would be midnight and the next day's pre-breakfast insulin would be only seven hours away, six hours earlier than if he/she had not left Sydney.

Conversely, people flying in a westerly direction would be going with the sun, extending the day and making the time between pre-breakfast insulins longer than if they had stayed at home.

This is probably not of great importance if the travel time between the Australian departure point and destination is less than four hours.

No person using insulin should undertake a long air flight without some basic information upon which he or she or the medical practitioner can make an intelligent decision about insulin dosage. Therefore, it is imperative to demand, some weeks ahead, that the travel agent obtain the information which can be used to put together a chart similar to the Chart on page 126.

Information required is the departure time, duration of flight, local time of arrival at each stop, time spent there before next take-off and the approximate time after each take-off when meals or snacks are served. This information is required for each leg of the flight – and don't be put off. The information is available so do not accept excuses. After all, why should some disinterested or uninformed person jeopardise your health?

Whether you are flying north, south, east or west, keep your watch on your home time and use this as a guide to when your insulin should be taken.

The dosage may require some adjustment in size or timing dependent on other factors during the flight.

Armed with the knowledge of the times of meals during the flight it should be possible to predict increases or decreases in dosage but in all cases these decisions must be checked by tests of blood sugar every two or three hours throughout the flight, with perhaps tests for the presence of ketones in the urine.

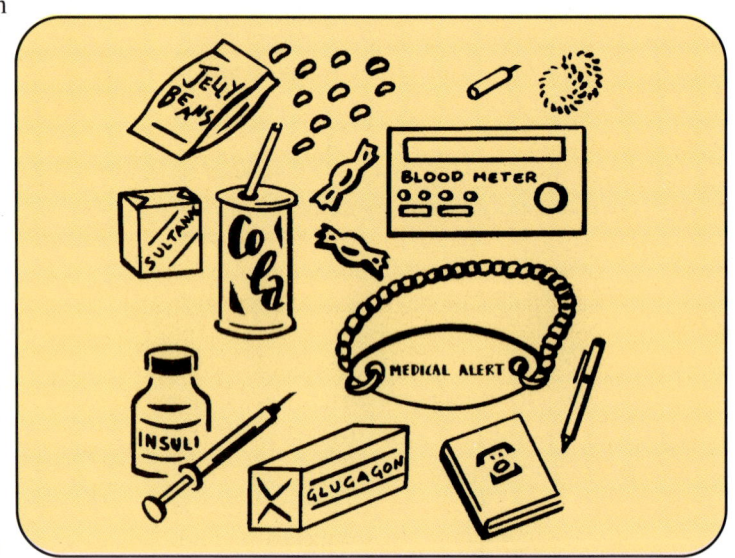

SURVIVAL KIT

Your 'SURVIVAL KIT' will deal with almost all problems of diabetes.
- *Quick acting carbohydrate, (eg glucose)*
- *Slow acting carbohydrate snack (eg dried fruits)*
- *Glucagon*
- *Quick acting insulin (neutral, clear)*
- *Blood testing equipment*
- *Medical alerting bracelet*

A single blood glucose estimation above normal would be no cause for alarm unless it was associated with the presence of moderate or heavy ketones – an unlikely event which would be an indication for immediate short-acting insulin.

A second or third moderately raised blood glucose level in the absence of ketones in the urine would be no cause for alarm if the routine insulin injection was to be taken shortly but if not, an extra injection of short acting insulin should be considered.

When considering whether to take extra short-acting insulin or not, the traveller should always bear in mind that hypoglycaemia in the air is not to be recommended. Safety is the key to success in the air – not perfect diabetic control. Therefore, adjustments to insulin or diet must be designed to avoid hypoglycaemia. Hyperglycaemia and/or ketoacidosis is highly unlikely to occur but hypoglycaemia may well occur in the patient who makes, or is advised to make, poorly considered dosage changes.

People who do not own a glucose meter should obtain some visually readable strips from Diabetes Australia or on prescription from their medical practitioner. These strips are easily read with the naked eye and people planning a trip should practice using them before they go. Branches of Diabetes Australia will advise the nearest Diabetes Education Centre where the procedure can be taught and if taking your own blood monitor: remember the spare batteries. People using insulin pumps or a basal long acting insulin once daily with small dosages of a short-acting insulin prior to the three main meals are unlikely to experience any great difficulties, regardless of the direction or duration of their flight. People on once or twice daily single or combined insulins will require changes, the complexity of which will differ depending on the normal daily dosage.

The most important point to remember is that if you are flying in an easterly direction and therefore having a shorter than normal day, you will require less insulin. If travelling in a westerly direction, you will require more insulin.

People flying to the east and therefore having their day shortened should reduce their morning intermediate or long-acting insulin by 20-30 per cent unless they also receive an intermediate or long-acting insulin prior to the evening meal, in which case this insulin should be reduced.

There will be occasions when the normal evening short-acting insulin dosage might also have to be reduced or even omitted altogether such as with people who have reached their destination at approximately midnight local time before the normal evening insulin was due. The same situation could apply to the person who was still en route eastward without any prospect of a meal within the next six hours.

Flights of less than four hours duration to the west would rarely require insulin dosage adjustment but those exceeding four hours extend the day and therefore the amount of food taken, meaning that insulin requirements would normally increase.

This is probably best achieved by giving an extra small dosage of short acting insulin, but an alternative could be to use intermediate acting insulin – the key being that in each case the maximum effect of the insulin must not occur when the person is asleep.

Insulin should never be taken until the meal is actually received or at arm's length. Arrival at the destination does not mean that the traveller may relax as either hypoglycaemia or hyperglycaemia could occur on that or the following day. The person may require extra short-acting insulin at unusual times throughout the day or night subsequent to arrival or alternatively, snacks to prevent hypoglycaemia produced by unexpected delays in customs or elsewhere.

Jet Lag

Jet lag is caused by a number of factors, particularly because our body's natural daily rhythm cannot change fast enough to keep pace with rapid changes from one time zone to another. It can be aggravated by lack of sleep, excessive alcohol and lack of exercise. A degree of exercise can be accomplished by walking up and down the aisle of the plane and walking, rather than sitting, in transit lounges during stopovers.

Even a few hours sleep is beneficial and this can be obtained by using suitable ear plugs obtainable from any pharmacy, plus a short acting sedative. The use of a sedative on the first few nights after arrival can also quicken the body's adjustment to the new time zone.

Sick Days

Chapter 13, Sick Days contains the essential elements needed by the traveller to care for himself or herself during an acute illness away from home.

Dried packet soups are not heavy or bulky and may be just the thing when the traveller is too ill to eat anything else. A small electric coil to heat broth, coffee or tea can be purchased from most electrical stores.

Remember that on sick days you must test your urine for the presence of ketones if you are insulin dependent. The presence of moderate or heavy ketones would be a very ominous sign and indicate the need for an urgent consultation. The casualty department of a hospital would usually be the source of the quickest and best treatment.

Blood and Urine Testing

The chapter on urine testing for glucose indicates that it has little role for people requiring insulin but it does have a place for some people whose diabetes is controlled by diet or diet plus tablets.

These people who do not require insulin should test more frequently than usual whilst travelling as the changed diet and exercise may result in either a marked improvement or deterioration in their diabetic control.

They should ask their doctor prior to departure what to do if there is sudden persistent increase or decrease in the amount of glucose in their urine.

People using a monitor should remember their machine may malfunction or be stolen on their travels and they should therefore practice visual reading of the strip for weeks prior to departure. When visual readout is not possible such as with Exactech, they should carry an emergency supply of BM 20-800 or Glucostix.

Medications

It has already been stated that all medications should be in double supply, with half in hand luggage and half in stowed luggage. The traveller should have a letter from a doctor stating his/her medications – including both the trade and generic names. The generic (or real) name will be useful in places where trade names differ to those used in Australia.

Diabetic people who use insulin should carry one or more ampoules of glucagon if they are travelling in remote areas of Australia or overseas. In the event of unconsciousness due to hypoglycaemia, consciousness should return within 15 minutes of glucagon being injected deeply into a muscle but if not, a second injection may be given.

The person accompanying the diabetic traveller should be well drilled in how to give an injection of glucagon, whilst a person prone to hypoglycaemia travelling alone should instruct another person, such as a flight attendant.

A sunscreen lotion may be required; insect repellents and particularly mosquito repellents in malarial areas; soluble pain killer for infants and an antibiotic ointment or a paint to treat cuts, blisters and the like.

Malaria is common in some countries and some forms of it may be fatal. The drugs used to treat or prevent malaria are effective but are themselves not without side-effects for some people.

It has been suggested that people who are visiting a malarial area for less than two weeks may not need to take anti-malaria treatment and furthermore that some drugs are best not given during pregnancy and breast-feeding.

Each traveller must discuss treatment with a medical practitioner or obtain advice from the Department of Health. The information is contained in Malaria Guidelines for Medical Practitioners which has been produced by the National Health and Medical Research Council of Australia.

Travellers' diarrhoea has been around so long it has been given quaint names like Delhi Belly and Montezuma's Revenge. These names suggest the condition is short lived and harmless,

Travel

which it is in the majority of cases, but not all.

Some cases cannot be self treated, such as when the diarrhoea includes blood in the bowel motion and a raised temperature. In such a case the patient requires medical attention.

However the majority of travellers with diarrhoea may undertake their own treatment, which should be in two stages. The first stage is to try to stop the symptom itself, namely the diarrhoea, without endeavouring to kill the organism responsible.

This is by use of drugs such as Imodium and Lomitil which suppress the contractions of the bowel and therefore stop the diarrhoea. They cannot be used for children under the age of 12 and an alternative in this case would be Kaomagma.

If the diarrhoea lasts longer than 48 hours drugs can be used to kill the organism responsible for the diarrhoea. This is the second stage. Bactrim, Resprim, Septrim are the trade names for a combination of two drugs used to treat a number of medical conditions including the organism responsible for traveller's diarrhoea and they can be used in patients of all ages.

Another effective treatment is Tetracycline or Doxycyline which cannot be used for children or during pregnancy or breast-feeding. Another drug for the treatment of traveller's diarrhoea is Norfloxacin. These drugs should be used for a period of not longer than five days and it should be remembered that they do not kill all organisms responsible for diarrhoea, for example, cholera.

Some people know from experience that they will develop traveller's diarrhoea every time they visit a certain country and it may be prudent to take low doses of these drugs throughout the period of their visit, providing it is not for longer than two or three weeks. The daily dosage for an adult is 100 mgs of Tetracycline or Doxycyline or one double strength tablet of Bactrim, Resprim or Septrim. All these medications for traveller's diarrhoea can have serious side-effects and the traveller must therefore seek medical advice before using them.

The fluid lost in the diarrhoea is an essential component of the human body and must be replaced or dehydration will certainly occur and this can lead to death in the very young or old. It is essential therefore that the traveller with diarrhoea takes adequate fluid replacement by mouth in the form of broths, or other sterile, non-alcoholic beverages.

Motion Sickness (Sea Sickness)

People with a past history of motion or sea sickness can lessen these symptoms by the use of Avomine (promethazine), Dramamine or Travacalm (dimenhydrinate) or Benacine (diphenhydramine). These drugs should not be used during pregnancy. They also can impair one's driving ability, especially if combined with alcohol.

❏ ❏ ❏

Travel is one of life's great joys. With planning and attention to detail, there is no reason why it should not be as enjoyable and rewarding for the person with diabetes as for anyone else.

> **TO WHOM IT MAY CONCERN**
> Re: Angela O'NEILL, Fitzroy Parade, FITZROY
>
> Angela O'Neill has Type 1 diabetes. She will have in her possession insulin, glucagon, syringes and equipment for testing the blood and urine for the presence of sugar. She will also have other medications including Oroxine (thyroxine).
>
> Her insulin dosage is Actrapid (Novo-Nordisk) 8-12 units prior to each meal with Humulin UL (Eli Lilly) 42 units at 10.00 pm.
>
> She is knowledgeable concerning the management of diabetes and it is unlikely that she will have any medical problems during her travel. However any requests for food or non-alcoholic drinks should be immediately granted.
>
> I would appreciate any assistance which you can give to my patient.
>
> Yours sincerely,
>
> DR C.M. THROUGH

CHAPTER 28

Further Resources

By Bernie Ayers
Director Health Promotion and Research
Diabetes Australia
Canberra

More than ever before the education, care and treatment needs of Australians with diabetes are being catered for by an ever increasing range of organisations, courses, products and education materials.

Having such a wide range of resources doesn't always make the task of choosing what is best any easier.

The key to learning more about diabetes is to look around and find those materials and learning tools which feel right for you, then use them as regularly as you can to achieve the best possible management of your diabetes.

Diabetes Australia—a good place to start

Diabetes Australia with offices in every capital city is the national organisation which represents and works for people with diabetes and their health professionals.

For more information contact any of the offices listed in this chapter direct or Diabetes Australia National Office, AVA House, 5/7 Phipps Place, Deakin 2600. Tel: (06) 285 3277; Fax: (06) 285 2881

The offices of Diabetes Australia are a good place to start when checking on available resources. Most State Associations of Diabetes Australia also have branches or regional networks which provide services to rural areas. They will be able to provide services and advice on a wide range of topics including:

- The latest in approved education and care leaflets, books, reports and videos. A national catalogue of education materials is now available through Diabetes Australia.
- Details on the Diabetes Australia National Diabetic Supplies Scheme for subsidised diabetic products (syringes and urine and blood glucose testing strips).
- The latest position on social issues, such as diabetes and driving.
- Advice on non or least discriminatory cover for life, travel, sickness and accident insurance.
- Advice on health care for those travelling interstate or overseas.

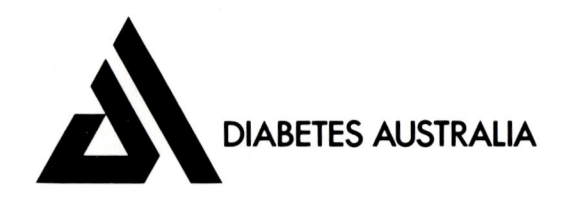

Most importantly, Diabetes Australia can:

- Provide access or referral to a range of other professional services, including dietary and podiatry services;
- Arrange camps or other self help meetings and activities where those with diabetes can share their experiences and feelings;
- Provide details on the availability of local resources and services.

You can become a member of Diabetes Australia for a small annual subscription and take advantage of all of these services. Membership also entitles you to a free copy of the national magazine, *"Conquest"*, as well as local newsletters and you will also be among the first to know of new publications such as this book. Educational materials are usually provided either free to members or at a substantial discount.

Further Resources

Another member organisation of Diabetes Australia, the Juvenile Diabetes Foundation – Australia, provides information, education materials and support services for those families who have a child with diabetes.

Hospitals, Clinics and Community Centres

Most major hospitals have diabetes centres or clinics which provide invaluable advice and support for persons who are newly diagnosed or for those who wish to stabilise their condition.

Many of these centres provide a complete range of services including medical, educational, dietetic, eye and foot-care. A number also run comprehensive courses for people with diabetes covering a range of topics similar to those included throughout this book. Another valuable facility offered by many of these clinics is a 24 hour hotline contact service.

Smaller hospitals and community health centres usually carry a more limited range of education materials but will know what services are available in their areas.

Doctors

Most general practitioners carry information on diabetes. Every general practitioner knows where further information and assistance can be found. Specialists in diabetes care, usually endocrinologists, carry a range of resource information and education materials and are very familiar with local services available in their areas.

Other Health Professionals

There may be times when you need to seek specific help and advice from a diabetes nurse, dietitian, pharmacist or podiatrist on a particular issue relating to diabetes management. Sometimes it may be appropriate to seek advice from the pharmaceutical company which supplies the diabetic aid or medication.

Never be afraid to ask for advice from any health professional. Because diabetes is so common in our community, most health professionals can provide advice and point you in the right direction for further information or for services you may require.

Bookshops and Libraries

The health sections of most bookshops and libraries stock books on diabetes.

A note of caution. The management of diabetes is a rapidly developing area of health with new technology and scientific updates occurring regularly. Books can date quickly. Those from overseas may also be confusing in their terminology and advice. It may be best to consult your doctor or diabetes nurse for advice before purchasing a book.

❑ ❑ ❑

NSW	149 Pitt St, Redfern 2016	Tel: (02) 698 1100
		Fax: (02) 698 4630
VIC	3rd Floor, 100 Collins St	Tel: (03) 654 8777
	Melbourne 3000	Fax: (03) 650 1917
QLD	Cnr Ernest & Merivale Sts	Tel: (07) 864 4600
	South Brisbane 4101	Fax: (07) 846 4642
SA	159 Burbridge Road	Tel: (08) 234 1977
	Hilton 5033	Fax: (08) 234 2013
WA	182 Bennett Street	Tel: (09) 325 7699
	East Perth 6000	Fax: (09) 221 1183
TAS	71 Davey Street	Tel: (002) 34 5223
	Hobart 7000	Fax: (002) 24 0105
NT	2 Tiwi Place	Tel (089) 27 8488
	Tiwi 0810	Fax: (089) 27 8515
ACT	GPO Box 149	Tel: (06) 247 5211
	Canberra 2601	Fax: (06) 257 6046
Juvenile Diabetes Foundation – Australia		
	PO Box 1500,	Tel: (02) 411 4087
	Chatswood, NSW 2067	Fax: (02) 411 8905

Where to look for help
- Diabetes Australia
- Local Hospital
- Community Health Centre
- Local General Practitioner
- Diabetes Nurse
- Local Pharmacy
- Bookshops and Libraries

DIABETES & YOU
An owner's manual

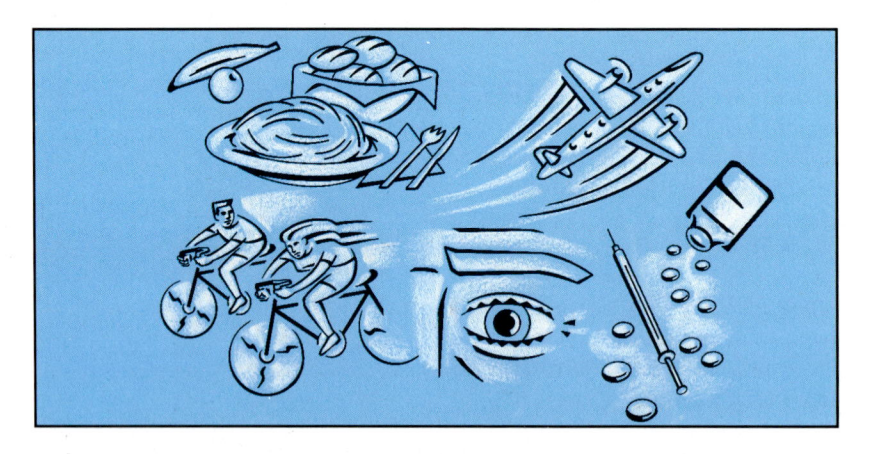

SPECIAL ISSUES

❏ The Genetics of Diabetes

Type 1 diabetes
Will my other children get diabetes
Type 2 diabetes

❏ Progress in Diabetes Research

The outlook for the future
Insulin gene therapy
Continuing progress in transplantation research
New methods of delivering insulin
Advances in Diabetes Research 1970 – 1990
Expected Benefits of Diabetes Research 1990 – 2010

CHAPTER 29

The Genetics of Diabetes

By Prof Susan Serjeantson
Professor and Head of Human Genetics
John Curtin School of Medical Research
Canberra

People with diabetes are obviously concerned at the chances of their children contracting diabetes. Just as common and understandable is the fear of parents with one diabetic child that their other children will also contract the disease.

In studying how diabetes runs in families, it is important to remember that Type 1 diabetes (insulin-dependent) and Type 2 diabetes (non-insulin dependent) are quite different diseases. In each disease the causes of high blood glucose are different.

Type 1 diabetes results from a process that destroys the insulin-producing cells of the pancreas. In Type 2 diabetes there is insulin, but the body is in some way resistant to its action. Given the clinical differences between Type 1 and Type 2 diabetes, it is not surprising to learn that they are caused by different genes.

Genetic factors are important in both types of diabetes. Studies of identical twins have shown this to be so. If an identical twin gets Type 1 diabetes, then the chance of the other twin getting diabetes is one chance in three, compared with about 4 per 1000 in the general population.

But just because the genes have predisposed diabetes does not mean people genetically at risk will automatically contract diabetes. In fact, two out of three identical co-twins do not get diabetes.

It is additional factors, such as viruses, trigger the disease in people who have the genes for Type 1 diabetes.

In Type 2 diabetes, if an identical twin gets diabetes, then it is very likely that the co-twin will also get the condition. The life-time risk to the co-twin is greater than 90 per cent. This means that in Type 2 diabetes genetic factors are more important than in Type 1 diabetes.

The two forms of diabetes are distinctly different clinical and genetic diseases, so must be considered separately.

Type 1 diabetes

In the mid-1970s, it was discovered that people with certain "HLA antigens" were more likely to get Type 1 diabetes than others.

The Human Leucocyte Antigens (HLA) are blood groups on white cells. In the same way that red cells have antigens, such as the ABO system, white cells also have antigen systems. The antigen systems of importance in Type 1 diabetes are called HLA-DR and HLA-DQ. In the ABO system, people can be blood group A, B, O or AB. A man who has the AB blood group has inherited the A gene from one parent and the B gene from the other. In the same way, the HLA genes are passed from one generation to the next, with each parent contributing one set of HLA genes to the child.

If a child inherits HLA-DR3 from one parent and HLA-DR4 from the other parent, their HLA type is DR3,DR4. This combination gives the highest risk for diabetes. If a child inherits HLA-DR2 from one parent and HLA-DR5 from the other, their HLA type is DR2,DR5 and they have almost no chance of getting Type 1 diabetes. The "high-risk" antigens for diabetes are HLA-DR3 and HLA-DR4, but, even so, by far the majority of people with these HLA types never develop Type 1 diabetes.

A recent study by Dr Glenys Thomson, an Australian working at the University of California at Berkeley, together with many international collaborators, compiled statistics from a large number of studies of families from

The Genetics of Diabetes

Australia, Europe and the US with Type 1 diabetes.

The study included nearly 1,800 people with Type 1 diabetes whose family members had been tested for HLA types. This is the largest set of data ever put together on Type 1 diabetes and now, more than ever before, an answer can be given to the question so often asked:

"Will my other children get diabetes?"

The overall chance for a brother or sister of a Type 1 diabetes patient developing Type 1 diabetes is 6 per cent or about 1 in 20. However, this overall figure masks the fact that some siblings have a low risk (1 in 75) while some have a much higher risk (1 in 5). This is because the actual risk for diabetes depends on the HLA types of the patient and that of the sibling.

If the patient has the HLA type DR3,DR4 and his sibling is also DR3,DR4, then the sibling has a risk for diabetes of 1 in 5 (19 per cent).

If the patient's sibling inherits neither DR3 or DR4 from his parents, then his risk for diabetes is only 1 in 50 (2 per cent).

If the sibling inherits one of the high risk HLA genes, then he also has a low risk (4 per cent). The diagram shows how HLADR types are inherited and how brothers and sisters of a patient can have different risks for Type 1 diabetes.

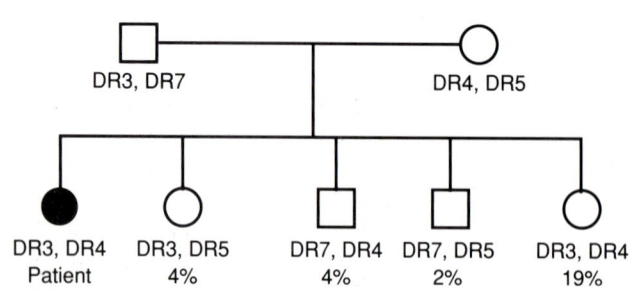

DR3, DR4	DR3, DR5	DR7, DR4	DR7, DR5	DR3, DR4
Patient	4%	4%	2%	19%

Risk for diabetes

Inheritance of HLA-DR types. Siblings of a Type 1 diabetes patient have different risks for disease, depending on their HLA-DR types.

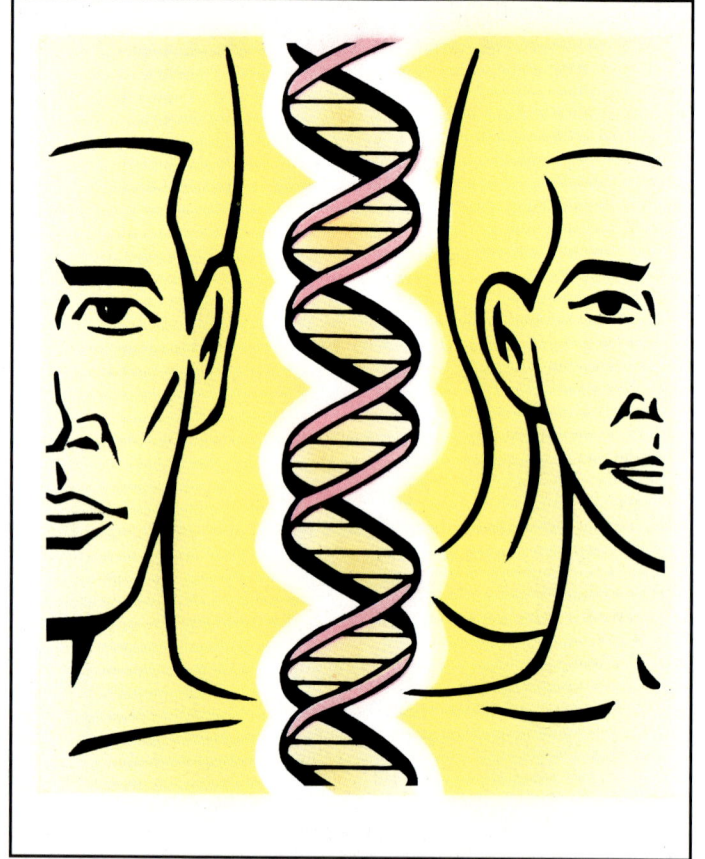

The precise risks for siblings of patients depend on the HLA types of both patient and sib. On average, if the patient and sibling have identical HLA types, the risk for the sib is 13 per cent. If the sibling shares one HLA antigen with the patient, the risk is 5 per cent. If the sibling has no HLA antigens in common with the patient, the risk is 2 per cent.

In one case in four, an unaffected brother or sister has HLA types identical with the patient. This means that in a family of five children, where one has Type 1 diabetes, one sibling will, on average, have a higher risk for diabetes (13 per cent) while the others will have a lower risk (2-5 per cent).

These figures can be reassuring to families where one child has Type 1

The Genetics of Diabetes

diabetes. If healthy parents of an affected child are considering another pregnancy, they can be assured that the risk for Type 1 diabetes in a subsequent child is about 1 in 20 (6 per cent).

The risks given here are life-time risks, calculated at birth. Clearly, the older the child, the less the risk for Type 1 diabetes. By the age of 20, the chance of getting the disease is negligible.

And so to the other most asked question: *"Will my children get diabetes?"*

Adults with Type 1 diabetes are obviously often concerned with the possibility of passing on the disease to any future offspring. The risk for children of a father with Type 1 diabetes is about 1 in 20 (6 per cent). There is a lower risk for children of a mother with diabetes. In one study, this risk was only 1 in 100 (1 per cent). Several studies have shown that children with a Type 1 affected mother may have some immunity to developing diabetes, but how this works is unknown.

When the father has diabetes, the risks for his children are once again dependent on the children's HLA types. There are low risks in some categories such as, for example, when the mother transmits the "resistant" DR2 type to the children. The highest risk is for DR3,DR4 children, where the chance of diabetes exceeds 1 in 5.

Of course potential parents are the ones to make the ultimate decisions and because individual cases vary, they may wish to obtain skilled advice from genetic counsellors. Counsellors will present the facts to the best of their ability, taking into account family history, HLA-types and so on. The parents can then consider the facts and decide whether to have children, or whether to have more children if one has Type 1 diabetes. Counsellors only provide the facts; the decision can only be the decision of the parents.

Type 2 diabetes

In Type 2 diabetes, the actual mechanics which cause the disease are unknown.

This is because diabetes causes so many disorders in sugar and fat metabolism, that it is difficult to pinpoint the primary defect among many secondary problems. Research is now concentrated at the genetic level, in order to define the basic inherited defects in the disease.

Candidate genes, including the insulin gene and the gene for the insulin receptor, have been examined in great detail at the molecular level. There are rare instances when defects in these genes cause diabetes, but usually in Type 2 diabetes these genes are quite normal. Attention is now focussed on genes encoding glucose transporters, the proteins that transport glucose into and out of cells. As yet the specific genetic defects have not been identified.

What is known is the risk to relatives of Type 2 diabetes patients.

There is a very high rate of concordance of diabetes in identical twins. If one twin develops Type 2 diabetes, the co-twin almost always develops the condition. The risk to siblings of Type 2 diabetes patients is about 30 per cent.

However, for Type 2 diabetes, even though a person may have inherited a tendency to develop diabetes, diet and exercise may postpone the onset of the condition, or diabetes may not develop at all.

There seems to be a "gene-dosage" effect in Type 2 diabetes – that is, when one parent has Type 2 diabetes, the chance of offspring developing diabetes is about 1 in 10 but if both parents have Type 2 diabetes, the chance of offspring developing diabetes is about 1 in 5. Likewise, the condition may develop earlier in people who have inherited two "diabetic" genes.

Type 2 diabetes is a mature-onset disease with the chance of developing it greater in older people. Indeed, the increase in prevalence of Type 2 diabetes in some populations may reflect an increase in life-expectancy.

For instance, in Caucasian populations, disease-onset is often at 60 years or older. In contrast, in high-risk groups such as Pacific Islanders, disease-onset is often at 40 years or older, with onset in 30-40 year olds not uncommon.

In some women with a tendency to diabetes, pregnancy can cause the condition to develop earlier than would otherwise be the case. In other

The Genetics of Diabetes

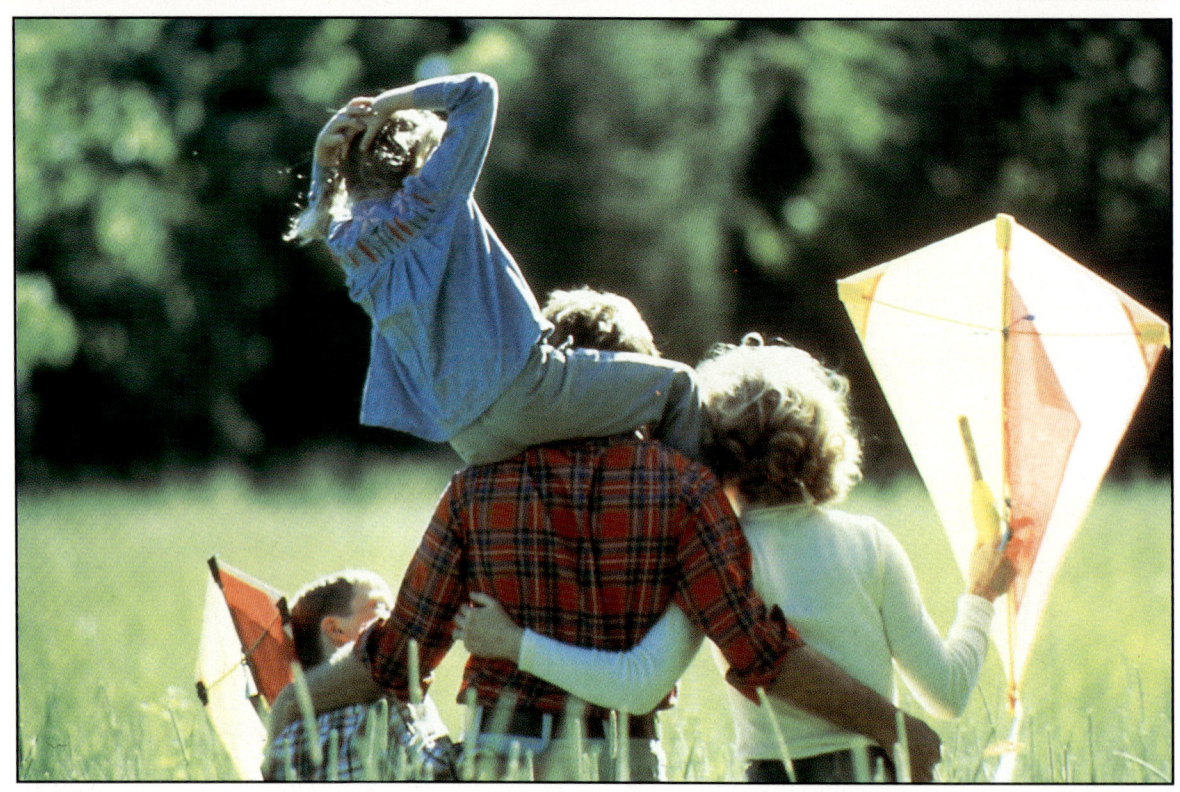

women, blood glucose levels rise during pregnancy, but these return to normal after the child is born. These women have demonstrated a tendency toward diabetes later in life. Women who have had gestational diabetes should have regular checks and do their best to adopt the healthy lifestyle that will keep diabetes at bay and under control.

Type 1 and Type 2 diabetes

There is, by chance, the occasional family with cases of both Type 1 and Type 2 diabetes. The diseases are, however, clinically and genetically distinct, with no interaction between the genes involved. Thus a family with cases of Type 2 diabetes has the same risks for Type 1 diabetes as the general population while relatives of a patient with Type 1 diabetes have the same risk for Type 2 diabetes as the general population. Therefore parents with a family history of Type 2 diabetes need not be concerned about passing Type 1 diabetes to their children.

CHAPTER 30

Progress in Diabetes Research

By Dr Kerry Bowen
Director, Diabetes Education Centre
Royal Newcastle Hospital, Newcastle
and Professor Leonard C. Harrison
Director, Burnet Clinical Research Unit
Walter & Eliza Hall Institute of Medical Research, Melbourne

Research and discovery in medicine does not usually proceed by "breakthroughs" but via a series of small steps and contributions from many scientists.

Eventually the final piece of the puzzle falls into place and **"Eureka!"**. This is how a new concept or a practical advance usually evolves and this process applies to diabetes research.

Even the pioneering experiments of Banting and Best which led in 1921 to the extraction of insulin from the pancreas of animals and the subsequent demonstration that injected insulin lowered the level of blood glucose in children with diabetes were preceded by similar experiments for almost 40 years.

But Banting and Best made it happen! Their treatment of diabetes using insulin injections was a life-saving advance in the treatment of Type 1 (insulin-dependent, juvenile-onset) diabetes. Giving insulin by injection does not cure Type 1 diabetes but it does enable many people with diabetes to live near-normal lives.

However, many will still develop the long-term complications of diabetes. These complications are thought to be due to the effects of a raised blood glucose over long periods of time, and the fact they still occur despite advances in our knowledge and the best usage of insulin indicates that there is a need to find a method of treatment which will return the blood glucose to the normal range for the 24 hours of each and every day.

At present, the only way to reliably achieve this goal is to transplant insulin producing cells into people who have diabetes. These cells are the beta cells which are found in the islets of Langerhans of the pancreas.

There are a number of ways by which this transplantation may be carried out. First, it is now possible to transplant the whole pancreas into people with diabetes. To do this successfully so that the transplant will function and produce insulin it is necessary to prevent the recipient from rejecting the foreign transplant.

Powerful drugs that suppress the immune system of the transplant recipient are required, but these drugs all have various side effects which may be quite severe at times.

As well the operation that is required is a major one, and so transplantation of the pancreas is not undertaken lightly. At present, any people with Type 1 diabetes who have developed kidney failure and require a kidney transplant are considered as possible candidates for pancreas transplantation.

A simpler way of transplanting the islet beta cells that produce insulin is to transplant the islets of Langerhans themselves. There are at least one million islets in the adult human pancreas and it has been estimated that at least 10% of these will be needed to reverse diabetes in humans.

Because they are so small the islets are readily transplantable by using fairly minor surgical procedures.

Therefore, the risk to the recipient from this form of transplant is slight when compared with that from transplantation of the whole pancreas. However, it is still very difficult to separate islets from the rest of the pancreas and therefore curing insulin-dependent diabetes by transplantation of islets has not yet become a practical proposition.

Nevertheless, it is very likely that the problem of obtaining sufficient islets for transplantation will be overcome within the next few years.

Progress in Diabetes Research

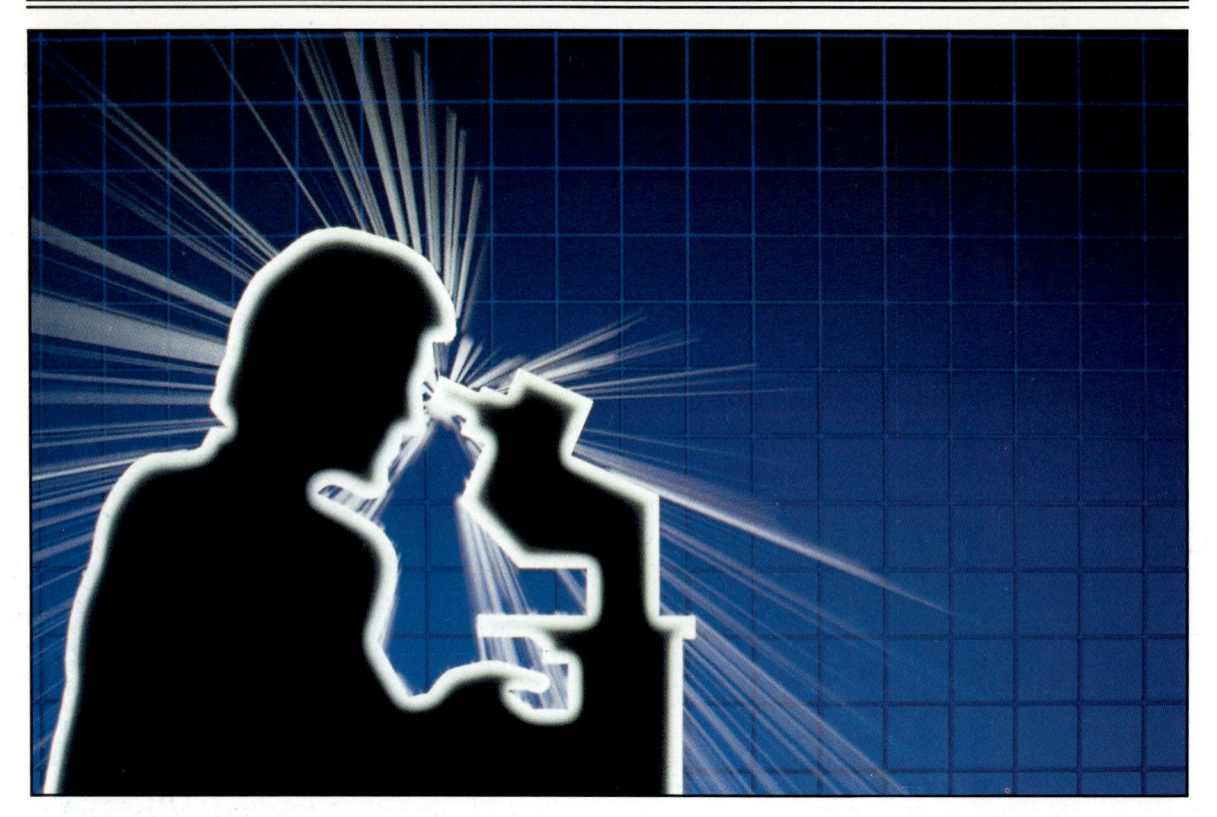

There have been many other advances in our understanding and management of diabetes over the last 20 years; these are detailed in table 1.

The outlook for the future

In the last 20 years there has been a tremendous increase in knowledge about the causes and effects of diabetes. The recent US study, The Diabetes Complication Control Trial, has shown that controlling diabetes does prevent or slow the progression of diabetic complications. There have also bee exciting advances in Type 1 diabetes, a disorder in which the immune system destroys the insulin-producing beta cells in the islets of Langerhans of the pancreas. What then lies ahead for the next 20 years?

Our current knowledge sets the scene for the early diagnosis and prevention of Type 1 diabetes, as well as providing for its cure in those who have already lost the ability to produce their own insulin.

In Type 2 (non-insulin dependent) diabetes mellitus, cells don't use glucose properly and are resistant to insulin, but the underlying cause(s) of this defect remain unknown. Nevertheless, we now understand much more about the way Type 2 diabetes is inherited.

We also know much more about the structure and function of important molecules such as the insulin receptor and the glucose transporter, which regulate how glucose is taken up and used by cells.

Insulin gene therapy

With the advances in genetic engineering techniques, scientists have been able to take the gene in the islet beta cell that programs the cell to make insulin and put this gene into other cells such as skin cells which can be grown easily in the laboratory.

This opens the way for insulin gene therapy. Using this technique, skin or bone marrow cells

TABLE 1: Advances in Diabetes Research 1970's – 1990's

Basic

- Family and population studies revealed the strong genetic transmission of Type 1 diabetes and the role histocompatibility (HLA) genes in predisposing to Type 1 diabetes.
- Type 1 diabetes was shown to be an autoimmune disease in which the body's immune cells (T and B lymphocyte cells) react against the islet beta cells as if they were foreign and eventually destroy them.
- The genes for several key protein molecules involved in glucose metabolism – insulin itself, the receptor for insulin on cells and the transporters for glucose within cells – were cloned, enabling these important molecules to be produced by genetic engineering.
- Techniques were developed to measure the metabolism of glucose in humans.
- Biochemical abnormalities were discovered in cells, that result from exposure of cells to high levels of blood glucose and which may lead to some of the chronic complications of diabetes.

Applied

- Methods were introduced for the self-monitoring of blood glucose.
- Purified animal insulins and genetically-engineered human insulin were introduced.
- New insulin delivery devices – pens and pumps – became available.
- Monitoring of chronic blood glucose levels by measuring glucose attached to proteins, eg. glycosylated haemoglobin, were introduced.
- The importance of high blood pressure in contributing to the blood vessel complications of diabetes was recognised and effective forms of treatment for high blood pressure were introduced.
- Risk factors for Type 1 diabetes, ie. family history, ethnic background, body weight, diet, diabetes in pregnancy and "stress" were recognised, and new approaches to the early diagnosis, prevention and treatment of Type 2 diabetes by attention to "life style" factors were adopted.
- The beneficial effects on the baby of controlling blood glucose levels in pregnant women with diabetes were clearly demonstrated.
- The advent of self-monitoring of blood glucose, pure insulin preparations and better means of administering insulin more frequently allowed many people with diabetes to achieve improved control of blood glucose.
- Significant advances were made in the monitoring and treatment of complications, eg. the introduction of angiography and laser treatment for diabetic retinopathy and kidney dialysis/transplantation for kidney failure secondary to diabetes.
- Specific drugs were developed, ie. the aldose reductase inhibitors, that block some of the effects of high blood glucose on cells.
- Transplantation of whole or segments of pancreas became practical and successful.
- The measurement of antibodies to the islet beta cells allowed individuals at high risk for developing Type 1 diabetes to be identified before the development of symptoms or insulin dependence.
- Treatment with drugs that suppress the immune system was shown to delay the progression to complete beta cell destruction in people with recent-onset of Type 1 diabetes.
- Based on knowledge of the immune mechanisms in Type 1 diabetes, specific forms of treatment were developed that prevent diabetes in animal models of the disease.

from a person with diabetes could be endowed with the ability to make insulin.

The major stumbling block here is finding how to 'transplant' not only the genetic machinery for making insulin but also that required for finely regulating its production in response to metabolic signals like glucose. There are many technical difficulties to be overcome but, given the rate of progress of genetic engineering, this almost ideal approach to replacing insulin may one day be feasible.

Continuing progress in transplantation research

Researchers have shown that diabetes in animals can be cured by the transplantation of pancreas obtained from foetal animals. Attempts have been made, therefore, to cure Type 1 diabetes in humans by transplanting pancreases obtained from aborted human foetuses, but so far without much success.

As with islet transplants, one problem is obtaining sufficient tissue, but with both islets and foetal pancreas the other problem is to ensure the tissue continues to live in the recipient.

Scientists are currently using animals to test the best site for transplanting islets and to discover substances (growth factors) that might stimulate transplanted islets to survive and function. The other avenue showing promise is the use of foetal tissue from pigs, which can be obtained in sufficient quantities and may be less likely to be rejected, thereby lessening the need for medications that suppress the immune system.

New methods of delivering insulin

As well as advances in transplantation, there are other exciting developments on the horizon. For example, eventually it may be possible to take insulin by mouth as ways are being developed to overcome the problem of orally ingested insulin being broken down by the digestive juices in the intestine.

Mechanical pumps designed to deliver insulin continuously to the body tissues have also been designed, and are becoming smaller and more refined year by year.

TABLE 2: Expected Benefits of Diabetes Research 1990's – 2010
• Environmental agents, eg. viruses or chemical toxins, that trigger Type 1 diabetes will be identified.
• Specific and safe forms of therapy will prevent the development of Type 1 diabetes in people in the pre-clinical stage of the disease.
• Specific forms of therapy will also be used to block rejection of islet transplants and the recurrence of autoimmune diabetes in transplants.
• Genetic engineering techniques for transplanting the insulin gene and its controlling mechanisms into a diabetic person's own cells, eg. skin cells, will be refined.
• The hi-tech artificial pancreas – a miniaturised insulin delivery pump connected to a non-invasive sensor for monitoring blood glucose – will be introduced.
• Oral medications will be designed or discovered that mimic the effects of insulin, as well as other medications that inhibit the effects of high blood glucose levels.
• Biochemical abnormalities in Type 2 diabetes that are inherited and cause cells to be defective in their use of glucose will be identified.

Overall, with the increasing amount of research into diabetes, it seems likely that the prevention, and possibly the cure, of Type I diabetes is nearing reality. Table 2 lists the likely benefits of diabetes research over the next 20 years.

❏ ❏ ❏

Glossary

Acetone: See ketone

Adrenal: A gland of the endocrine system that produces essential hormones including adrenaline and cortisone.

Albumin: A water soluble protein present in the urine with kidney damage (albuminuria).

Alpha Cells: Cells in the pancreas that produce the hormone glucagon.

Angiography: A rapid series of pictures of blood vessels made after a dye has been injected.

Antibodies: Substances occurring naturally in the body that help fight infection.

Arteriosclerosis/Atherosclerosis: Thickening, hardening and narrowing of the arteries.

Artery: A blood vessel that carries blood away from the heart.

Aspartame: A low calorie artificial sweetener.

Beta Cells: The insulin producing cells of the pancreas.

Callus: A hardened or thickened part of the skin caused by pressing or rubbing.

Calorie: A measure of the energy value of foods (now replaced by kilojoule: 1 calorie = 4.2 kilojoules.

Candida: A yeast like fungus infection often affecting the female genital area.

Capillary: Tiny blood vessels that connect the smallest arteries to the smallest veins.

Carbohydrate: Foods which contain sugars and starches.

Cardiovascular: Pertaining to the heart and blood vessels.

Cataract: An opacity in the lens of the eye.

Cell: The microscopic unit that forms the basis of all living things.

Cholesterol: A fatty substance produced by the human body and also found in animal tissue.

Claudication: Pain in the calf muscles occurring on exercise and disappearing with rest. Caused by decreased blood supply.

Coma: Loss of consciousness from any cause. In diabetes from very high or very low blood glucose levels.

Creatinine: A waste product normally removed by the kidneys.

Cyclamate: A low calorie artificial sweetener.

Cystitis: An inflammation of the urinary bladder.

Glossary

Dehydrated: Loss of water or fluid from the body.

Dextrose: See glucose.

Dialysis: Artificial removal of waste products from the blood when the kidneys fail.

Digestion: Breaking down food in the stomach and intestines.

Electrocardiograph:(ECG) The recording of the electrical activity of the heart.

Endocrine Glands: Glands that produce chemicals (hormones) which affect other body cells.

Enzyme: A substance that speeds up a chemical reaction.

Exchanges: Servings of food that contain the same food value. Also known as portions.

Fat Atrophy/Hypertrophy: Hollows (atrophy) or lumps (hypertrophy) that occur at sites of repeated insulin injection.

Fibre: Food substances found in cereals, fruits and vegetables that are not digested but help the function of the intestines.

Fluorescein: A harmless yellow coloured dye that is used to outline the vessels of the eye.

Fructosamine: A glycated protein like glycated haemoglobin that measures glucose control over the preceding weeks.

Fructose: A sugar found in fruits.

Gangrene: Death of body tissue usually caused by lack of blood supply.

Gestational: Referring to the period of pregnancy from conception to birth.

Glomerulus: A tiny tuft of blood vessels that is part of the functional unit of the kidney.

Glucagon: A hormone produced in the pancreas that increases blood glucose.

Glucose: The form of sugar found in the human body.

Glucose Tolerance Test: A diagnostic test for diabetes involving a drink of glucose and a series of blood glucose estimations.

Glycated/Glycosylated Haemoglobin: Haemoglobin with glucose chemically bound to it.

Glycosuria: The presence of glucose in the urine.

Haemoglobin: The red coloured iron protein that carries oxygen in red cells.

Glossary

Haemoglobin A1C:	See glycated haemoglobin.
HLA:	Human leucocyte antigens which are natural markers on white cells much the same as blood groups on red cells.
Hormone:	A chemical substance produced by endocrine glands which causes specific effects on other cells.
Hyperglycaemia:	Blood glucose higher than normal.
Hypertension:	High blood pressure.
Hypoglycaemia:	Blood glucose level lower than normal.
Impotence:	The inability in males to start, sustain or complete the act of sexual intercourse.
Insulin:	A hormone produced by the pancreas that lowers blood glucose.
Insulin Dependent Diabetes:	See Type 1 diabetes.
Intramuscular:	Administration of a medication through a needle into the muscles.
Intravenous:	Administration of a medication through a needle into a vein.
Islet Cell (of Langerhans):	Clusters of cells in the pancreas which include the beta (insulin producing) and alpha (glucagon producing) cells.
Juvenile Onset Diabetes:	See Type 1 diabetes.
Ketones:	Chemical substances from the breakdown of fat which can be dangerous in large amounts.
Ketones in the Urine (Ketonuria):	Warns of ketoacidosis.
Ketoacidosis:	Uncontrolled blood glucose and ketone levels that cause dehydration, concentration of body fluids, build up of acids (acidosis) and coma.
Kilojoule:	A measurement of the energy of food which has replaced calorie (1 calorie = 4.2 kilojoules).
Lactic Acidosis:	A serious condition caused by the build up of lactic acid which is produced from glucose when there is not enough oxygen. Similar effects as ketoacidosis.
Lactose:	A sugar found in milk.
Laser (Light Amplification by Stimulated Emission of Radiation):	An intense narrow beam of light which can be used to heal damaged areas in the body (e.g. blood vessels in the eye).

Glossary

Macrovascular:	Referring to the large blood vessels.	Photocoagulation:	Use of the laser to treat diabetic eye disease.
Maturity Onset Diabetes:	See Type 2 diabetes.	Plasma:	The liquid portion of blood.
		Polyuria:	The passage of large amounts of urine.
Metabolism:	The physical and chemical changes occurring in the body.	Portions:	See exchanges.
Microalbuminuria:	Leakage of small amounts of protein (albumin) into the urine. An early warning of kidney damage.	Prandial:	Referring to meals e.g. pre-prandial: before meals; post-prandial: after meals.
		Pruritus:	Itching.
Microvascular:	Referring to the small blood vessels.	Renal Threshold:	The blood glucose level above which glucose spills into the urine.
Millimole (mmol):	A measurement of the concentration of chemicals in the body.	Retinopathy:	Damage to the retina of the eye.
Monilia:	See Candida.	Saccharin:	A low calorie artificial sweetener.
Nephropathy:	Disease of the kidneys.		
Neuropathy:	Disease of the nerves.	Somogyi Effect:	A rebound effect of low followed by high blood glucose caused by too much insulin.
Non Insulin Dependent Diabetes:	See Type 2 diabetes.		
		Sorbitol:	A sugar used to sweeten foods.
Obesity:	The condition of severe overweight.	Subcutaneous:	Underneath the skin.
Oral Hypo-glycaemic Agents:	Medications taken by mouth that stimulate the release or improve the action of insulin.	Sugars:	Simple carbohydrates which are sweet and occur widely in nature e.g. fructose, glucose, lactose, sucrose.
Pancreas:	A gland lying towards the back of the abdomen half way between the tummy button and line joining the nipples.	Sucrose:	A common widely available sugar from sugar cane or sugar beet.

Glossary

Thrush: See Candida.

Thyroid: An endocrine gland in the base of the neck producing hormones controlling the body's metabolism.

Triglyceride: A type of fat found in the blood and other parts of the body.

Type 1 Diabetes: Where little or no insulin is made, usually occurring under the age of 30 and requiring insulin injections for life. Also known as insulin dependent and juvenile onset diabetes.

Type 2 Diabetes: Insulin is present but doesn't work adequately. Usually occurs over the age of 30 and is controlled by diet and medication or diet and insulin. Also known as non insulin dependent and maturity onset diabetes.

Unit: The measurement of the dose of insulin.

Uraemia: Build up of poisons because of kidney failure.

Vein: A blood vessel that carries blood to the heart.

For a listing of health professionals see Chapter 21 "You and Your Health Care Team".

Index

A
Aborigines 112
    diet 113
    incidence 112
    prevention 114
    reversal 113
Alcohol 12, 19

B
Blood Glucose 39
Blood glucose monitoring 2, 6, 39
    frequency of testing 40
    how to test 40
    inaccurate results 43
    influencing factors 40
    lancets 43
    measurement range 40
    meters 42, 44
    strips 41
Blood pressure 75, 100
Blood vessel disease 76
Breakfast 20

C
Carbohydrates 15
    complex 11
Cataract 75, 82
Children 105
    food 108
    hypoglycaemia 106
    ketoacidosis 108
    physical problems 105
    psychological problems 108
Childrens' camps 37, 108
Cholesterol 56
    HDL 56
    LDL 56
Clinics 7, 133
Coma 51
Complications 75
    blood vessel disease 76
    eye damage 75
    hypoglycaemia unawareness 78
    infections 77
    kidney damage 77
    nerve damage 77

D
Diabetes
    diagnosis 6
    gestational 92
    Type 1 5, 135
    Type 2 5, 137
Diabetes Australia 8, 132
Diet 15
    on sick days 64
Dining out 19

E
Eight golden guides 11
Emotions 95
Energy 15
Ethnic communities 110
Exercise 11, 56, 99
    aerobic (v) anaerobic 61
    extra carbohydrates 58
    foot problems 60
    how much 61
Eyes 81, 100, 118
    examinations 81
    eye damage 75, 81
    poor eyesight and injections 37
    laser treatment 83
    malculopathy 83
    ophthalmologist 81, 101
    retinopathy 81

F
Fat
    atrophy 35, 79
    hypertrophy 35, 79
    invisible 18
    monounsaturated 18

Index

polyunsaturated	18	hollows	35
saturated	18	lumps	35
visible	18	method	34
Feet	86, 103	side effects	35
foot care	86	site for injection	33, 103, 118
foot first aid	88	Injectors	32
footwear	87	automatic	37
nerve damage	84	jet	37
podiatrist	86, 101	pen	36
Fibre	16	Insulin	25, 127
		allergy	79
G		beef	27
Gene therapy	140	dose	127
Genetics	135	human	27
Type 1	135	intermediate acting	27, 30
Type 2	137	long acting	27, 30
Gestational diabetes	92	mixed	27, 30
Glucagon	53	porcine	27
Glucose	6	problems	29
Glycaemic index	17	short acting	27, 30
Glycated haemoglobin	91	storage	28
Golden guides	4, 11	strength	27
Groceries	19	types	27, 30
		uses	27
H		Insulin dependent diabetes	
Health care team	99	(see Diabetes Type 1)	
High blood glucose		Insurance	120
(see hyperglycaemia)		advice	122
Hyperglycaemia	2, 51	influencing factors	122
causes	54	information required	121
symptoms	53	health & travel	123
treatment	54		
Hypoglycaemia	2, 51	**J**	
causes	51	Jellybeans	52
children	106		
symptoms	51	**K**	
treatment	52	Ketoacidosis	62, 108
unawareness	53, 78	Ketones	47
		Kidney damage	77, 102
I			
Injections	32		
age	37		
bruising	35		

Index

L
Lancets	43
Life insurance	120
Lifestyle	11
Low blood glucose (see hypoglycaemia)	
Lumps	35, 79

M
Meals	19, 64
Medications	68, 99
blood glucose level	68
insulin response	71
urine glucose	71
Meters	
buying a meter	42
models available	42, 44
Migrant communications	110
Migrant health services	110
Monitoring	
health care team	99
responsibilities	99
see blood glucose monitoring	
urine glucose testing	

N
National Diabetic Supplies Scheme	100, 132
Needles	32
Nerve damage	77
Nephropathy	77
Neuropathy	77
Non insulin dependent diabetes (See Diabetes Type 2)	

O
Ophthalmologist (see eyes)	81, 101

P
Pancreas	3, 6
transplant	142
Podiatrist (see feet)	86, 101
Pregnancy	89
common concerns	91
complications	92
gestational diabetes	92
pre-existing diabetes	89
Proteins	18

Q
Quit for life	12

R
Renal threshold	46
Research	135, 139
Retinopathy (see eyes)	75, 81
Resources	132
Responsibilities	117
Rights	117

S
Sexual problems	
erections	96
men	96
treatment	96
women	95
Sick days	62, 130
diet	64
extra insulin	63
food and drink	64
ketoacidosis	62
monitoring	62
travel	130
vomiting	66
Starches	15
Stress	11
Strips	
blood glucose	41
care of strips	42
temperature	127
urine	47
Sugars	15, 52
Superannuation	122
Syringe	32

Index

T
Tablets	69
effectiveness	21
side effects	21
when ill	22
Take 30	22
Take time out	11
Team approach	99
Travel	123
blood and urine testing	130
documents	123
insulin	127
insulin dosage	127
insurance	123
itinerary	123
jet lag	129
medication	130
motion sickness	131
sick days	130

U
Urine glucose testing	46
interpretation	49
medications	71
recording results	49
renal threshold	46
testing for glucose	47
testing for ketones	47
testing for protein	48
when to test	48

W
Weight	15, 99, 118

XYZ
Xanthoma	79
Xanthelasma	79

Abbreviations & Measures

Abbreviations

cc	cubic centimetre
cm	centimetre
g	gram
kg	kilogram
L	litre
mg	milligram

mmol = millimole
  (eg: 5 mmol/L = 5 millimoles per litre)
Kj   Kilojoule
Cal Calorie

Measures

1 level teaspoon = 5 ml
1 level tablespoon = 20 ml
1 cup = 250 ml

1 Kj = 1000 joules
1 Cal = 4.2 Kj
1 oz = 28.4 g;
1000 g (1 kg) = 2.2 lbs

1 pint = 570 ml
1 fluid oz = 28.4 ml;
1000 ml (1 litre) = 1.76 pints

Diabetes and You – An owner's manual represents more than 12 months work involving 30 of Australia's leading experts in the field of diabetes education and care.

Diabetes Australia sees the manual as its official text and reference source on diabetes education and care issues. A series of publications based on the manual have also been produced.

Every person with diabetes should have a copy of this manual for ready reference as part of their day to day management routine.